Building Blocks for Primary Prevention

Protecting Children from Lead-Based Paint Hazards

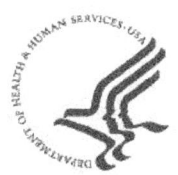

October 2005

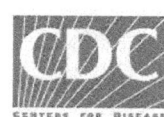

Building Blocks for Primary Prevention: Protecting Children from Lead-Based Paint Hazards

Centers for Disease Control and Prevention

NATIONAL CENTER FOR ENVIRONMENTAL HEALTH

LEAD POISONING PREVENTION BRANCH
Mary Jean Brown, ScD, RN, Chief

Produced by the Alliance for Healthy Homes, Washington, DC

October 2005

Suggested reference:
Building Blocks for Primary Prevention: Protecting Children from Lead-Based Paint Hazards. Atlanta: CDC, 2005

TABLE OF CONTENTS

BUILDING BLOCKS FOR PRIMARY PREVENTION

EXECUTIVE SUMMARY

This publication offers a comprehensive collection of 70 "building blocks," which are primary prevention strategies that merit consideration by state and local governments and others in position to reduce exposure to hazards in housing and thereby help meet the Healthy People 2010 goal of eliminating childhood lead poisoning. Exemplary strategies span a broad spectrum which includes targeting high-risk properties; widely instituting safe work practices; building community capacity to check for hazards and work safety; delivering hazard assessment, control and prevention services; motivating action; screening high-risk housing; expanding financial resources; strengthening enforcement; raising public awareness and support; and establishing valuable partnerships. A strategy has been considered for inclusion as a building block if it is sensitive to the economics of affordable housing, consistent with the principles of public health, holds the potential for broad-scale impact, stands a reasonable possibility of implementation, and offers promise for reducing lead and other environmental health hazards in high-risk housing. The summary of each building block is coupled with an illustration of how the strategy has been implemented and contact information for at least one individual who is knowledgeable about this activity. The purpose of disseminating *Building Blocks for Primary Prevention: Protecting Children from Lead-Based Paint Hazards* is to allow programs and policymakers easy access to information about innovative and promising strategies that span the spectrum of primary prevention, from which they may select one or several to pursue based on their jurisdiction's needs and political and economic realities.

INTRODUCTION

Context and Background

Exposure to lead continues to poison young children in the United States. Estimates based on data from 1999 and 2000 indicate that about 2.2% of children aged 1-5 years (about 434,000 children) have blood lead level (BLL) elevations at or above 10 micrograms per deciliter ($\geq$10 μg/dL). *Healthy People 2010* (Objective 8-11)[i] calls for the eradication of lead poisoning as a public health problem by the year 2010 through the elimination of elevated blood lead levels in children.

Over the past decade, research has greatly expanded understanding of the sources and pathways of lead exposure in the residential environment and the effectiveness of a range of strategies to make housing safe. While children can be exposed to lead from a variety of other sources and pathways, the most significant cause of exposure is the presence of lead-based paint hazards in their homes, such as lead in non-intact paint, interior settled dust, exterior soil and dust, and hazards created by improperly conducted renovation work. Focus on the presence of lead-based paint and its lead content has given way to recognition of the importance of the condition of painted surfaces in older homes and the dangers of lead-contaminated dust. Chronic ingestion of settled lead dust on floors, windowsills, and other surfaces is now recognized as the foremost pathway of young children's exposure to lead in the home environment, and dust lead levels are recognized as the strongest predictor of risk.

Based on the recommendations of an interagency working group tasked with planning to achieve the 2010 lead elimination goal, the *Federal Strategy for Eliminating Childhood Lead Poisoning*[ii] emphasizes the essential need to require action before children are poisoned—by making the US housing stock lead-safe. The latest national survey of lead hazards in US housing makes clear the magnitude and complexity of this challenge: more than one-quarter of all US housing units pose "significant lead hazards."[iii]

Yet the impact of most lead poisoning prevention programs is limited to the fraction of properties that are occupied by a child with an elevated blood lead level (less than two percent of hazardous units nationwide). While the need continues to improve blood lead screening and case management services, achieving the national 2010 goal of eliminating lead poisoning as a public health problem requires significantly increasing the impact of primary prevention strategies to make high-risk housing lead-safe.

The Centers for Disease Control and Prevention (CDC) has a longstanding responsibility and commitment to protecting children from lead poisoning. Since the early 1970s, CDC has made grants to help state and local health department lead poisoning prevention programs screen children at risk for lead poisoning or elevated blood lead levels (EBL), perform environmental investigations to determine the source children's exposure, and provide follow-up case management and educational services. At the national level, CDC works closely with other federal agencies committed to lead poisoning prevention, notably the US Department of Housing and Urban Development's Office of Healthy Homes and Lead Hazard Control (HUD OHHLHC), the US Environmental Protection Agency (EPA), and, within the US Department of Health and Human Services, the Centers for Medicare and Medicaid Services (CMS) and the Office of Community Services (OCS).

The Lead Poisoning Prevention Branch of CDC is fulfilling its commitment to the 2010 lead elimination goal through its grant program's requirement that jurisdictions develop and implement a strategic plan for elimination that includes primary prevention, partnering, and program evaluation. Through this *Building Blocks* publication, the Branch now offers grantees and others access to a compendium of promising primary prevention approaches to reduce exposure to lead paint hazards.

State and local childhood lead poisoning prevention programs (CLPPPs) universally acknowledge the importance of primary prevention and are beginning to address it in their strategic plans and funding applications. However, many programs' primary prevention efforts are confined to parent education about hygiene, nutrition, and housekeeping, despite research that makes clear the limitations of these interventions for families whose homes pose significant lead hazards. Inability to institute durable primary prevention is caused in part by the pressure to focus resources and attention on secondary prevention by identifying and managing individual cases of elevated childhood blood lead level (BLL). Indeed, in communities where follow-up on actual poisonings is limited to educating family members about lead hazards and behavioral change (because public resources are not available to control identified lead hazards and halt further exposure), meaningful primary prevention can seem like an extremely remote target. Programs facing these circumstances need ideas for sharing responsibility within the jurisdiction to stop repeat offenders, expand access to lead-safe housing, and ultimately arrest the cycle of inferior housing that continually produces new poisonings.

While no city or state with a significant stock of leaded housing has successfully assembled all of the elements needed to make primary prevention a reality across the jurisdiction, state and local lead poisoning prevention programs across the country and their partners in other agencies and the private sector have implemented a multitude of innovative and successful primary prevention strategies over past years. Workshops and conferences periodically feature model programs, but the prospect of replicating an entire program with multiple components and elements can be daunting to the CLPPP seeking to evolve beyond screening and case management. Difficulty in achieving program transformation to primary prevention is only compounded within an overwhelmed public agency that is surrounded by a change-resistant or risk-averse political environment. Since most successful primary prevention programs consist of multiple elements, specific strategies can be considered individually or in combination.

The multitude of innovative strategies to identify, control, and prevent lead hazards in housing before a child is poisoned that are currently being implemented across the country has never been systematically documented or described in a way that makes information about their design and implementation readily accessible. Programs and their jurisdictions need this information at the "building block" level in order to decide which strategies to pursue based on local needs and conditions. This document identifies and describes individual building blocks across the spectrum of primary prevention strategies in order to create access to knowledge about tangible and realistic opportunities for progress and program evolution in identifying, controlling, and preventing lead poisoning and other housing-related health hazards.

Scope and Limitations

The research for *Building Blocks for Primary Prevention: Protecting Children from Lead-Based Paint Hazards* was guided by the descriptions of primary prevention in CDC's 1997 screening guidelines and 2002 case management guidelines, which emphasize eliminating and controlling toxic exposures at the source. While primary prevention necessarily encompasses activities that address all sources of exposure to lead, this publication is focused on strategies for preventing and controlling lead hazards in housing, the foremost cause of poisoning.

A strategy has been considered for inclusion as a building block if it is sensitive to the economics of affordable housing, consistent with the principles of public health, holds the potential for broad-scale impact, has a reasonable possibility of implementation, and offers real promise for reducing lead and other environmental health hazards in high-risk housing. Building blocks are not only technical tools and program elements but also strategies such as techniques for targeting high risk housing, leveraging opportunities, innovative partnerships, enforcement mechanisms, expanded financial resources, and new ways to bring lead safety and healthy homes tools into broader use. A building block is more likely to be a key ingredient of a prevention-based system, rather than an entire program.

The heart of the challenge to public health agencies is leveraging action to make privately owned housing lead-safe. Many CLPPPs are increasingly viewing leveraging action to address lead hazards in housing as a part of their leadership role. While public health program directors and staff are clearly the primary audience for *Building Blocks*, some strategies entail fostering change in other organizations and systems to advance prevention in high-risk housing. The summary of each building block is coupled with an illustration of how the strategy has been implemented and contact information for at least one individual who is knowledgeable about this activity.

Building Blocks has some inherent limitations that deserve note. The information listed in illustrations (partners, resources, constraints) is not comprehensive but rather a citation of specific and strong examples of building blocks. Results of efforts to replicate a given building block will vary depending on individual state and local laws, maturity of partnerships, political will, and the existence and strength of community-based partners. The applicability of a building block selected for implementation will depend on the maturity and capacity of the jurisdiction and its CLPPP. Inclusion of building blocks in this document does not assure that they have been evaluated for their outcome or transferability.

Organization of Building Blocks
The description of each strategy reflects the template **(Appendix A)** that has shaped the research and compilation of *Building Blocks*. The generalized information includes the title, brief summary, potential applications and benefits (including scope of impact), and critical elements such as staffing patterns, other resource needs, institutional capacity, cost and timing considerations, and indication of feasibility of implementation.

At least one real-world illustration amplifies building block descriptions by documenting the scope and particulars of the example in a given jurisdiction or target area; the staffing and other resources utilized; magnitude of its impact; factors essential to implementation; limitations encountered; estimated potential for replication; and specific contact information and references for additional information. The illustrations offer strong examples of how each strategy has been recently implemented but do not provide an inclusive or exhaustive review of all efforts to ever plumb the benefits of the given strategy.

This document displays building blocks grouped by the category that best fits their essential contribution:
- Building Awareness and Public Support
- Building Capacity for Lead Safety
- Collaborations, Partnerships, and Incentives
- Financing and Subsidies
- Lead Safety and Healthy Homes Standards
- Targeting High-Risk Homes
- Using Code Enforcement and Other Systems

An alphabetical index of of the building blocks follows the Introduction.

The internet edition of *Building Blocks for Primary Prevention: Protecting Children from Lead-Based Paint Hazards* will be available in Summer 2005 through the website of the Lead Poisoning Prevention Branch, www.cdc.gov/nceh/lead. Through this site, it will be possible to easily select sections of Building Blocks for online review and search by keyword, location of illustration, category, key actor or partner, and similar criteria.

ACKNOWLEDGEMENTS

Members of the Advisory Committee on Lead Poisoning Prevention and countless individuals working in local and state programs contributed many valuable ideas, feedback, and real-world illustrations.

The team that researched and wrote *Building Blocks* under CDC's contract with the Alliance for Healthy Homes, headed by Project Director Jane Malone, included Nick Farr, Laura Fudala, Brian Gumm, Carol Kawecki, Jane Malone, Betsy Marzahn-Ramos, Gordon McKay, Tom Neltner, Anne Phelps, Eileen Quinn, Maria Rapuano, Don Ryan, Ralph Scott, Ellen Tohn, Anne Wengrovitz, and Anne Ziebarth.

The CDC Lead Poisoning Prevention Branch's Chief Mary Jean Brown, Philip Jacobs, Rob Henry, and numerous other staff of the Lead Poisoning Prevention Branch contributed important guidance and feedback at critical junctures in the development of *Building Blocks*.

---

[i] Healthy People 2010: understanding and improving health. US Department of Health and Human Services. Washington, DC: 2000.

[ii] Eliminating Childhood Lead Poisoning: A Federal Strategy Targeting Lead Paint Hazards. President's Task Force on Environmental Health and Safety Risks to Children, Washington, DC: 2000.

[iii] National Survey of Lead and Allergens in Housing, Volume One, Westat for the US Department of Housing and Urban Development and National Institute for Environmental Health Sciences, 2001.

ALPHABETICAL INDEX OF BUILDING BLOCKS

BUILDING AWARENESS AND PUBLIC SUPPORT

ANALYZE AND PUBLICIZE DATA TO FACILITATE IMPROVED POLICIES

CREATE A "DEMONSTRATION HOME" TO EDUCATE POLICY MAKERS AND THE PUBLIC

CREATE AND USE MULTI-STAKEHOLDER ASSESSMENTS AND REPORTS TO ADVOCATE FOR PREVENTION

ENGAGE RENTAL PROPERTY OWNERS ON LEAD SAFETY, DISCLOSURE, AND OTHER RESPONSIBILITIES

EXPAND LEAD SAFETY EDUCATION TO EXPECTANT AND NEW PARENTS

INTEGRATE LEAD POISONING PREVENTION EDUCATION INTO PHYSICIAN EDUCATION CURRICULA

ORGANIZE "TOXIC TOURS" FOR POLICY MAKERS

PUBLICIZE PROBLEM RENTAL PROPERTY OWNERS

PUBLICIZE RESTRICTIONS ON UNSAFE REMODELING AND RENOVATION

USE DATA FROM COMMUNITY HOME HAZARD INVESTIGATIONS TO ADVOCATE FOR POLICY SOLUTIONS

USE INVESTIGATIVE JOURNALISM TO REVEAL DIMENSIONS OF THE PROBLEM AND POLICY SHORTCOMINGS

ANALYZE AND PUBLICIZE DATA TO FACILITATE IMPROVED POLICIES

DESCRIPTION OF THE STRATEGY

Communities can generate greater awareness and improve targeting of resources by analyzing and publicizing data to highlight geographic patterns and other information about lead poisoning and asthma.

Because citywide averages, although useful in many respects, tend to camouflage disparities in risk of lead poisoning or asthma, small area analysis is a critical component of this strategy. In small area analysis, communities "drill down" beyond the municipal level and analyze data for smaller geographical areas. The most telling analysis would examine data by census block or neighborhood, but parsing data by ZIP code is also illuminating. Unlike a citywide average, these levels of analysis can identify concentrations, or "pockets," of lead poisoning and asthma, allowing regulators, property owners, and community-based organizations to focus attention and resources.

Detailed data analysis will be most effective when the data are presented using clear and compelling visual aids, such as color-coded maps. Several organizations have found that a great way to leverage data to improve policies is to show prevalence rates by political jurisdiction (e.g. by city council district). Mapping data in this way focuses the attention of city council members whose districts are home to concentrated pockets of lead poisoning and asthma. Residents of high prevalence areas can use the information to mobilize their neighbors to secure policy improvements.

BENEFITS

Immediate/Direct Results: This strategy produces useful, detailed information in a format that allows the public and decision makers to recognize geographic disparities in lead poisoning prevalence and risk and know where to target the most aggressive risk reduction efforts.

Public Health Benefits: Identifying areas with the highest risk can prompt more immediate action to prevent lead poisoning by targeting code enforcement and lead hazard control efforts where most needed within a jurisdiction.

Other Indirect/Collateral Benefits: Graphical representations of disparity data can spark discussion and increase resolve to address other issues related to those disparities: urban blight, poverty, substandard housing, and more. It can also encourage better policies that assist both targeted areas and the municipality as a whole.

SCOPE OF POTENTIAL IMPACT

City- or County-Wide   Neighborhood/Community

PRIMARY ACTORS

Community-based Organizations

KEY PARTNERS

Health Department
Human Services Agency
Tenants
Parents
Community Members

CRITICAL ELEMENTS

Staff requirements: Projects using this strategy are generally short-term but time-intensive. In some organizations and agencies, existing staff can perform the data analysis and presentation; others may need temporary help from experts in data analysis and/or mapping.

Other resource requirements: Access to lead screening data that includes addresses and zip codes will be required. Mapping and graphics software and knowledge of political jurisdiction boundaries (council districts, legislative districts within or including a particular municipality, etc.) are also essential.

Institutional capacity required: Command of data analysis and mapping software is essential to successful implementation of this strategy.

Cost considerations: Moderate costs will be incurred if outside consultants are needed. Costs for software, handouts, flyers, and other publications can be expected.

Timing issues: For maximum impact, results should be made public to policy makers as they are weighing key decisions, such as annual budget allocations or new policy proposals.

Feasibility of Implementation: High. Past successes have shown that this strategy is replicable in other jurisdictions. Free or minimal cost options could be explored to make this strategy even more replicable. Local programs could request support from state agency partners, and states could ask for support from CDC or other federal agencies. Alternatively, agencies may be able to tap into government-wide information technology resources, borrow staff from other agencies with expertise in mapping software and small area analysis, or utilize functions of existing programs.

POTENTIAL OBSTACLES/BARRIERS

Perhaps the most significant potential obstacle is a lack of knowledge or skill, particularly when it comes to specialized mapping skills and GIS software. However, partnering with other organizations with such knowledge or contracting out for such skills can overcome this obstacle.

Other barriers could include a lack of responsiveness from policy makers or the absence of sufficient lead poisoning data by zip code or census block. Care must be exercised to protect the confidentiality of medical information.

ADDITIONAL RESOURCES
N/A

ILLUSTRATION #1 OF STRATEGY IN PRACTICE

In 2002, Philadelphia Citizens for Children and Youth (PCCY) issued a report, "Un-Leaded Only: Toward A Safer City For Children," documenting ongoing lead hazards and poisoning problems throughout the city of Philadelphia.

As part of that report, PCCY used a small area analysis conducted by the Philadelphia Department of Public Health's Childhood Lead Poisoning Prevention Program (CLPPP). This analysis looked at childhood poisoning data by ZIP code and then overlaid that information to city council boundaries. The result was a map included within the PCCY report that showed a striking range of poisoning cases. The data showed 51 cases of childhood lead poisoning in Council District 10, and 872 cases in Council District 3 in 2001. The data also showed that for children living in the city's highest risk zip codes, the rate of elevated lead levels is more than ten times higher than the national average.

Jurisdiction or Target Area: Philadelphia

Primary Actor: Philadelphia Citizens for Children and Youth, Philadelphia Dept. of Health's Childhood Lead Poisoning Prevention Program

Secondary Actor(s): N/A

Staffing utilized: The Philadelphia CLPPP estimates that one person-day was used in creating the map. The data used had already been coded and was stored in an excellent "front-end" database. Organizations and health departments looking to replicate this strategy should be aware that automating data in a format usable for such analysis may take substantially more time depending on the condition of the database.

Other resources utilized: ArcView software, a Council District map, and the "front-end" database were all utilized in producing the lead poisoning map.

Factors essential to implementation: CLPPP staff knowledge of small area analysis and utilizing mapping software was critical. The ability of CLPPP and PCCY to partner to present the data as part of a larger report allowed for the information to be widely distributed and widely reported by the media.

Limitations/challenges/problems encountered: No significant problems or challenges were encountered.

Magnitude of Impact/Potential Impact: The map included in the PCCY report supported the authors' assertions that lead poisoning remains a serious problem in Philadelphia. It also provided a striking graphic representation of disparities of risk within the city, which captured the attention of the media and policymakers alike.

Potential for replication: The potential for replication of this strategy is high if staff time and mapping software is available and cooperation with local or state health authorities exists.

Contact for Specific Information:

Richard Tobin
Director
Philadelphia Childhood Lead Poisoning Prevention Program
215-685-2788

Colleen McCauley
Health Care Projects Manager
PCCY
215-563-5848 x33
colleenmccauley@pccy.org

References for additional information:
1. PCCY, "Un-Leaded Only: Toward A Safer City For Children"
    www.pccy.org/PDF/Lead%20Report.pdf

ILLUSTRATION #2 OF STRATEGY IN PRACTICE

In 2002, the New York Public Interest Research Group (NYPIRG) used data from the health department to issue a report about childhood lead poisoning disparities in New York City. This study was conducted in conjunction with a campaign to pass the new lead poisoning prevention law in New York City that was enacted in February 2002.

NYPIRG was aware that while the number of children poisoned by lead in New York had been declining for years, there appeared to be stubborn pockets of poisoning throughout the city, particularly in low-income neighborhoods. NYPIRG conducted a small area analysis of the data—they first analyzed the data by census block and then aggregated it by ZIP code. The analysis confirmed that there were indeed concentrated pockets of childhood lead poisoning in New York, many of which were located in low-income areas with tracts of substandard housing.

In order to convince City Council members that the existing lead poisoning prevention policy was not working for all of the city's children, NYPIRG decided they needed to illustrate the extent of the disparities in New York by converting the ZIP Code data to the corresponding city council districts. The resulting map showed the concentration of lead poisoning in each council district.

NYPIRG, in conjunction with the New York City Coalition to End Lead Poisoning, released the data at a press conference, almost immediately drawing support for the city's new lead poisoning prevention law from several additional council members.

Jurisdiction or Target Area: New York City

Primary Actor: New York Public Interest Research Group (NYPIRG) and the New York City Coalition to End Lead Poisoning (NYCCELP)

Secondary Actor(s): N/A

Staffing utilized: 1.5 FTE for several weeks.

Other resources utilized: ArcGIS, ArcView, and other mapping software.

Factors essential to implementation: Access to the mapping tools and to the data from the health department were both critical, as was NYPIRG's commitment and capacity to support the project in the absence of dedicated grant funding.

Limitations/challenges/problems encountered: NYPIRG had to file a Freedom of Information Law (FOIL) lawsuit to obtain the lead poisoning data from the state health department at a reasonable cost and in a useable format; the department initially wanted to charge 25 cents per page of data.

Magnitude of Impact/Potential Impact: The presentation of the small area analysis data by city council district had great power and enormous impact as demonstrated by the level of support the new lead poisoning prevention law received. The law eventually passed and survived a mayoral veto.

Potential for replication: The potential for replication of this strategy is high if funding and staff time is available. Any CLPPP can pursue this strategy. CBOs need to secure data from health departments, either cooperatively or by filing a Freedom of Information Act (FOIA) request.

Contact for Specific Information:
Pete Sikora
New York Public Interest Research Group
212-349-6460
psikora@nypirg.org

References for additional information:
1. Goldberg and Palmer, NYPIRG, "Do You Know Where the Lead Is?"
   www.nypirg.org/lead/whereslead/
2. Community Mapping Assistance Project, Technical Resources
   www.cmap.nypirg.org/about_cmap/resources.asp

CREATE A "DEMONSTRATION HOME" TO EDUCATE POLICY MAKERS AND THE PUBLIC

DESCRIPTION OF THE STRATEGY

Just as homebuilders use model units to give a prospective buyer a vivid sense of the home they might purchase, lead poisoning prevention advocates can create "demonstration homes" to show how lead paint hazards can develop and demonstrate techniques for controlling lead hazards, as well as highlighting other healthy homes problems and solutions in a powerful way. The demonstration home can include hands-on, interactive components to provide a wide range of important and practical facts about lead poisoning prevention. Advocates can partner with key stakeholders to create and operate the demonstration home and invite policy makers and opinion leaders to tour the home, opening doors for further collaborations and discussions about needed policy changes.

BENEFITS

Immediate/Direct Results: This activity immediately provides practical education about lead hazards and lead safety to all who participate in its development, as well as to those who visit the home. It demonstrates to trades people and policy makers alike that many techniques for identifying and reducing lead paint hazards are simple and affordable, and provides an opportunity to explore the nuances of what interventions are appropriate for various circumstances.

Public Health Benefits: This demonstration vividly teaches policy makers that lead safety can be achieved in many cases through interventions that are lower cost than typically believed. It also dramatically illustrates why lead-safe work practices and lead dust clearance testing are vital—and realistic—activities when old paint is disturbed.

Other Indirect/Collateral Benefits: By working together to create and operate the demonstration home, key stakeholders (such as tenant groups, homebuyers, affordable housing advocates, health care providers, hardware and paint stores, unions, building trades people, and do-it-yourself remodelers) build a foundation for deeper collaborations on lead poisoning prevention.

SCOPE OF POTENTIAL IMPACT

By inviting elected officials, agency staff, housing court judges and prosecutors, reporters, and other policy makers and opinion leaders to tour the home, advocates can open doors for further partnerships and discussions about needed policy changes.

City- or County-Wide   Neighborhood/Community

PRIMARY ACTORS	KEY PARTNERS
Health Department	Code or Building Inspection Agency
Community-based Organizations	Housing Agency
	Child Welfare Agency
	Family Services Agency
	Property Owners
	Tenants
	Contractors
	Painters
	Equipment Suppliers and Retail Stores
	Utility Companies
	Parents
	Homeowners

CREATE A "DEMONSTRATION HOME" TO EDUCATE POLICY MAKERS AND THE PUBLIC

CRITICAL ELEMENTS

Staff requirements: Depend upon the goals and features of the demonstration home. One half-time person working with other volunteers could create a basic version of this in 2-3 months. The schedule for visitors could be limited to specific dates and times to minimize staffing requirements.

Other resource requirements: Basic equipment and materials that might be helpful for demonstrating lead safety techniques include lead spot tests, lead dust testing supplies and materials, HEPA vac and other cleaning supplies, photo displays of "before and after" conditions, photos or other graphics documenting the process of hazard remediation using different approaches, and take-home materials.

Institutional capacity required: People creating the demonstration home must be familiar with a wide range of lead safety techniques and interventions and know relevant laws that guide acceptable practices. Anyone engaging in hazard identification or remediation practices should have all required credentials.

Cost considerations: This can be a very cost-effective way to reach key audiences with practical information, generate press coverage, and influence policy. The dwelling unit, equipment, materials, labor, and other in-kind items can be solicited from local real estate or housing development organizations, hardware/home improvement stores, labs, and community groups. If successful, another institution (government agency, store, health clinic, etc.) might agree to assume responsibility for maintaining the demonstration home in the future.

Timing issues: In the northern United States, warmer months are best for creating the home and attracting visitors.

Feasibility of Implementation: High. Partnerships with agencies and organizations that can play a constructive role are key for success.

POTENTIAL OBSTACLES/BARRIERS

Finding an easily accessible home that can be used for a substantial period is the major challenge. The impact of the strategy depends on drawing policy makers and other visitors to the demonstration home.

ADDITIONAL RESOURCES
N/A

ILLUSTRATION OF STRATEGY IN PRACTICE

In Spring 2003, the Get The Lead Out Project created a "lead lab" for two months in a vacant house that was built in 1894. The project documented extensive lead hazards and low-cost hazard control treatments, and then conducted tours and open houses for officials and others. Various "stations" in the house featured basic lead poisoning information, photos documenting creation of the lead lab house, lead-safe cleaning tools, lead-safe work practices brochures and materials, dust wipe sampling kits, and an XRF machine. Project members demonstrated a variety of window treatments to reduce lead hazards, ranging from well liners to window replacement. A portable blood lead analyzer allowed people to have their own blood lead levels checked. Visitors took a lead dust wipe sample in the house. Visiting the demonstration home motivated several state and local officials to engage with advocates in substantial ways on subsequent policy and program matters. Local residents, property owners, code enforcement officers, and city officials became more aware of the problems of lead hazards and options for addressing them.

Jurisdiction or Target Area: Rochester, NY

Primary Actor: Orchard Street Community Health Center's Get The Lead Out Project

Secondary Actor(s): Environmental Health Sciences Center, Dept. of Environmental Medicine, University of Rochester; Monroe County Department of Public Health HUD Lead Hazard Control Grant Program

Staffing utilized: Coordinator documented approximately 0.6 FTE, supplemented by volunteer contractors, risk assessors, outreach, etc.

Other resources utilized: HEPA vacs, XRF analyzer, portable blood lead analyzer, dust sampling kits, cleaning tools/supplies, photos of conditions and hazard control procedures. Recommend photo and video documentation.

Factors essential to implementation: Partnerships among local agencies, owners, neighborhood group.

Limitations/challenges/problems encountered: Short life span of project.

Magnitude of Impact/Potential Impact: About 100 visitors in one month. Entire project was done for very low cost. More visitors could have been drawn if demonstration home were to be maintained for a longer period.

Potential for replication: High. The extent of the program depends on local partners and constraints.

Contact for Specific Information
Katrina Korfmacher
Community Outreach Coordinator
585-273-4304
Katrina_Korfmacher@URMC.Rochester.edu

References for additional information
N/A

CREATE AND USE MULTI-STAKEHOLDER ASSESSMENTS AND REPORTS TO ADVOCATE FOR PREVENTION

DESCRIPTION OF THE STRATEGY

By conducting and publicizing a local or regional assessment of the status of lead poisoning prevention and screening efforts, policies, and barriers, advocates can develop a community-wide agenda with concrete action steps to address identified needs. Such assessments and subsequent action plans can best be written by a "task force" that represents the major stakeholders who will need to be engaged to carry out the plan—including: health and housing agencies, code agencies, community and health advocates, property owners, and others.

BENEFITS

Immediate/Direct Results: The assessment can pull together and communicate a clear picture of the scope of the problem and the reasons that underlie the status quo. It can identify opportunities and barriers to instituting primary prevention and vet models from other jurisdictions that should be considered. Involving multiple stakeholders in the assessment process fosters a common understanding of the problem and a shared basis for considering possible solutions. Stakeholders who have committed to investigating the problem become invested in implementing solutions. Ideally, the assessment will clarify specific roles of stakeholders and hold them accountable for implementing aspects of the resulting strategy.

Public Health Benefits: The assessment process can build public and political support for a clearly described approach and expand resources for preventing and controlling lead hazards in housing as well as other sources.

Other Indirect/Collateral Benefits: This process can build working relationships and cooperation among different stakeholders that can be tapped for tackling other community problems.

SCOPE OF POTENTIAL IMPACT

Statewide—Assessment can lay groundwork for new state legislation
Regional (e.g. multi-county)
City- or County-Wide

PRIMARY ACTORS

Health Department
Housing Agency
Community-based Organizations

KEY PARTNERS

Code or Building Inspection Agency
Human Services/Medicaid Agency
Child Welfare Agencies
School Districts
Property Owners
Tenants
Contractors
Painters
Retail Stores
Equipment Suppliers
Physicians
Hospitals
Parents

CRITICAL ELEMENTS

Staff requirements: The coalition or agency coordinating the assessment needs to include people with experience in a broad array of disciplines, including affordable housing, landlord-tenant issues, the construction trades, real estate finance, code enforcement, and leaders of affected communities. The assessment can help broaden support by involving all pertinent government agencies (health, housing, code enforcement, and social services), elected officials, and key private sector individuals who need to be part of the solution (e.g. landlords, contractors, health care providers). All participants do the key work on a shared, in-kind basis, although staffing a successful process could take as much as one FTE during periods of intense activity.

Other resource requirements: To create a common basis for decision-making, the assessment should compile and analyze data that clarifies the problem, including lead poisoning rates and exposure patterns as well as key housing variables—*e.g.* housing age, type of construction, occupancy, and rental ownership patterns. The assessment should also analyze relevant laws, regulations, codes, ordinances, and other important factors in the legal and policy landscape. This analysis should go beyond lead-specific laws, such as lead-safe housing standards, blood lead screening requirements, and contractor certification systems, to consider all relevant sections of housing, sanitary, and building codes and landlord-tenant laws, the extent of lead poisoning tort litigation, and agencies' regulatory powers.

Institutional capacity required: Top management support to convene and carry out assessment process.

Cost considerations: Cost of staff for administrative support and legal research.

Timing issues: The assessment should map out the windows of opportunities for implementing recommendations, and how and when stakeholders need to weigh in to influence policymaking. For example, the results of a purposeful assessment will inform and determine public agency strategy planning, regulatory decisions, passing new legislation, and annual budget decisions.

Feasibility of Implementation: High

POTENTIAL OBSTACLES/BARRIERS

The budget shortfalls in many jurisdictions can discourage participants who fear there will be no resources to devote to the recommendations that could emerge. The assessment can address this by looking for innovative financing mechanisms.

It is possible that the dynamic of the process encourages participants to pursue idealistic proposals that would not be enforceable or are out of step with market conditions in the jurisdiction. The process needs to bring together data and research that will ground the deliberations of the assessment participants and whenever possible, investigate how potential policies have been implemented in other communities.

ADDITIONAL RESOURCES
N/A

ILLUSTRATION OF STRATEGY IN PRACTICE
The Lead Safe Pittsburgh Coalition is a multi-stakeholder coalition that is designing a regional assessment to define the lead poisoning problem. The Coalition will use the policy paper resulting from this assessment to build community and political support for solutions and as a blueprint for future efforts. The Coalition plans to use a consultant to help compile the data, conduct disinterested interviews with stakeholders, analyze the policy landscape, and identify model policies from other jurisdictions.

Jurisdiction or Target Area: Allegheny County/greater Pittsburgh area

Primary Actor: Lead Safe Pittsburgh Coalition

Secondary Actor(s): N/A

CREATE AND USE MULTI-STAKEHOLDER ASSESSMENTS AND REPORTS TO ADVOCATE FOR PREVENTION

Staffing utilized: The coalition is expending 0.3 FTE and is conducting monthly meetings of staff from represented agencies.

Other resources utilized: Consultant.

Factors essential to implementation: The broad membership in the Lead Safe Pittsburgh Coalition is a critical factor that portends a successful assessment; members include business interests, financial institutions, broad representation from public interest organizations, and agency staff from city and county health and housing organizations. It has the capacity to attract additional stakeholders and considerable relevant expertise to bring to bear on the multi-faceted aspects of the problem.

Limitations/challenges/problems encountered: Budget problems in Pittsburgh and the state will pose considerable challenges to the coalition's efforts to build support for solutions. Moving to primary prevention will likely require passing new state legislation to mandate primary prevention and update existing lead certification program requirements. Finally, most of the recommendations will need to be implemented by government agencies. The Coalition is grappling with the challenge of how to establish accountability among the stakeholders, so that government actors will be accountable to the rest of the participants for implementation.

Magnitude of Impact/Potential Impact: The Coalition anticipates achieving changes in state legislation and has been building a relationship with advocates in other parts of the state, most notably Philadelphia Citizens for Children and Youth.

Potential for replication: High. This strategy is one that could be adopted elsewhere, at the local, county, regional, or state level. In fact, government agencies and public interest organizations are pursuing this approach in Rhode Island, Chicago, and Boston, among other locations.

Contact for Specific Information
Moira Singer
Director, Lead Safe Pittsburgh Coalition
412-431-4449, ext 205
moiras@ccicenter.org

References for additional information
N/A

ENGAGE RENTAL PROPERTY OWNERS ON LEAD SAFETY, DISCLOSURE, AND OTHER RESPONSIBILITIES

DESCRIPTION OF THE STRATEGY

Proactively engaging area landlords is an innovative way to build public awareness and support vital to advancing lead poisoning prevention and healthy housing. Health departments and community-based organizations can foster less adversarial, more supportive relationships with landlords by combining presentations of traditional lead prevention information with subjects that landlords see as being in their self-interest. Such topics can include free training in lead-safe work practices; how hazard control interventions can reduce legal liability; sources of grants and loans for rehabilitation and lead abatement; and information about other services such as low-cost clearance testing.

BENEFITS

Immediate/Direct Results: Landlords will become better informed about lead hazard prevention and control, lead-safe work practices, and services available to them that make controlling and abating lead hazards more affordable. Good working relationships will also be established among health departments, landlords, and community-based organizations, which can help encourage broad action to reduce and eliminate lead hazards.
Public Health Benefits: Landlords who are aware of practical lead poisoning prevention tools and resources will be less likely to inadvertently create lead hazards through rehabilitation or remodeling, and they will be better equipped to control existing lead hazards.
Other Indirect/Collateral Benefits: Good working relationships with landlords can be used to encourage these property owners to incorporate further healthy homes practices on their properties.

SCOPE OF POTENTIAL IMPACT

City- or County-Wide   Neighborhood/Community

PRIMARY ACTORS	KEY PARTNERS
Health Department	Housing Agency
Community-based Organizations	Rental Property Owners/Landlords

CRITICAL ELEMENTS

Staff requirements: 0.5 FTE at the most; in most instances, no new staff will be required.

Other resource requirements: Prior contacts with already-cooperative landlords can be useful to this strategy.

Institutional capacity required: This strategy builds on existing laws and programs.

Cost considerations: Modest costs can be expected, and overall costs will depend on the scope of the strategy.

Timing issues: This strategy can be implemented at any time.

Feasibility of Implementation: Variable. Feasibility will largely depend on landlord response to engagement efforts.

POTENTIAL OBSTACLES/BARRIERS

In some areas, landlords may continue to be resistant to change or cooperative working relationships with government regulators and/or community-based organizations, despite persistent efforts to engage them. In other instances, landlords may deem necessary efforts "too expensive," setting up adversarial relationships this strategy is supposed to avoid.

ADDITIONAL RESOURCES

N/A

ILLUSTRATION OF STRATEGY IN PRACTICE

As part of a larger lead hazard investigation and policy project, the Greensboro Housing Coalition decided to directly engage area landlords on controlling existing lead hazards, lead-safe work practices, and other healthy housing issues.

The Coalition invited landlords to attend a series of free dinners. The dinners allowed landlords to get to know Coalition staff and community members personally and presented a wide variety of useful information on lead hazards, potential liabilities, responsibilities of property owners, and more.

Jurisdiction or Target Area: Greensboro, North Carolina

Primary Actor: Greensboro Housing Coalition

Secondary Actor(s): N/A

Staffing utilized: 0.5 FTE on a limited-term basis was needed to plan and hold the dinners.

Other resources utilized: N/A

Factors essential to implementation: The main factor essential to the implementation of this strategy was the interest of landlords in the dinners. Other factors that helped make the strategy a success included the city's commitment to reducing lead hazards and improved vigilance in holding landlords accountable for health hazards in their properties.

Limitations/challenges/problems encountered: Some landlords were completely uninterested in the dinners. There was also some contention at the dinners over the Coalition's practice of conducting lead hazard investigations at no charge to tenants without landlords' knowledge or prior approval. However, discussion of this issue proved useful, as it illustrated the need for ongoing communication between property owners and healthy housing advocates.

Magnitude of Impact/Potential Impact: 38 landlords attended the dinners, and 12 more, though unable to attend, requested the information packets distributed at the dinners.

Potential for replication: This strategy holds a high potential for replication. While the dinners did require a significant planning and organizational effort, they were not extremely staff-intensive. In communities where landlords are eager to reduce their potential liabilities or where lead hazard enforcement has been steadily increasing, this strategy should prove extremely useful.

Contact for Specific Information

Beth McKee-Huger
Executive Director, Greensboro Housing Coalition
336-691-9521
beth@greensborohousingcoalition.com

References for additional information

1. Greensboro Housing Coalition
   www.greensborohousingcoalition.com/

EXPAND LEAD SAFETY EDUCATION
TO EXPECTANT AND NEW PARENTS

DESCRIPTION OF THE STRATEGY

Educational initiatives can be used to inform pregnant women of the danger of lead-based paint and lead dust hazards and are especially important in high-risk areas. Enhanced education and outreach programs to expectant and new parents can include information about lead poisoning, evaluation and control of lead hazards, home preparation, local lead safety resources and community groups, and screening recommendations. Indeed, educational programs can offer tangible support for primary prevention, such as vouchers for classes in lead-safe work practices or even cleaning equipment.

BENEFITS

Immediate/Direct Results: Each woman who learns about lead hazards may be motivated to take actions to reduce lead exposure to herself, her infant, and other family members. Reaching expectant and new parents is true primary prevention.

Public Health Benefits: Broad and sustained community-wide education targeted to expectant and new parents can yield changes in collective behavior and understanding. In particular, community norms about controlling lead hazards in the home or otherwise preparing the home for newborn children may be changed over time, creating more lead-safe homes and benefiting more families including children of all ages.

Other Indirect/Collateral Benefits: Increased community-wide awareness can generate broad commitment to improve community resources and political will for primary prevention.

SCOPE OF POTENTIAL IMPACT

Statewide

City- or County-Wide

Regional (e.g. multi-county)

Neighborhood/Community

PRIMARY ACTORS

Health Department

KEY PARTNERS

Medicaid Agency

Physicians

Expectant Parents

Housing Agency

Head Start

WIC

Community-based Organizations

CRITICAL ELEMENTS

Staff requirements: Varies, depending on the extent of the initiative and existing parent education activity (if any) by the sponsoring entity.

Other resource requirements: Appropriate mechanisms for delivery and dissemination of desired educational messages are needed, but the mechanisms can vary dramatically depending on the design of the educational initiative. Typical educational methods include brochures, fact sheets, and web sites. The considerable range of materials already developed on lead safety obviates the need to develop materials, although modifications should be made to incorporate local referral resources. Programs can augment traditional materials with more attention-getting vehicles, such as diaper bags and other promotional items. Any materials used must be accessible and understandable to those who live in high-risk areas, where language barriers and reading levels can present a challenge. Programs will also need data and surveillance information.

Institutional capacity required: Health education initiatives rarely require special authorization.

Cost considerations: Adding a new subject to an existing education program is more cost-efficient than implementing free-standing education focused only on lead safety. Printing materials will cost nominal amounts per parent.

Timing issues: Can be implemented anytime

Feasibility of Implementation: Variable. Feasibility depends on the availability of people to manage the effort and resources to support it.

POTENTIAL OBSTACLES/BARRIERS

One potential obstacle is reaching agreement on a specific strategy deemed most effective for the circumstances, as there are so many possible combinations of messages, messengers, delivery mechanisms, and possible target audiences. In addition, it can be uncomfortable to make lead-safety recommendations to parents in communities where resources do not exist to assist families in repairing lead hazards.

A barrier to the effectiveness of education on lead safety is the fact that expectant and new parents may already be overwhelmed with other recent messages on multiple weighty issues and have many other concerns and priorities. Discussion of possible lead exposure *in utero* may help parents to focus attention on the immediacy of lead safety.

Programs may also encounter unexpected challenges in developing partnerships with seemingly natural partners. For example, one program reported difficulty in convincing obstetricians to participate in such an educational campaign.

ADDITIONAL RESOURCES

N/A

ILLUSTRATION #1 OF STRATEGY IN PRACTICE

MA CLPPP conducted a project to educate pregnant women about lead hazards and encourage them to adopt preventive behaviors, and to educate doctors and staff members for community health centers and agencies in the target communities. The project's three core activities were:

1. Development and distribution of bilingual prenatal lead awareness kits packaged in large attractive diaper bags. The kit included educational fact sheets and brochures, promotional items, a community resource card, an evaluation card, and a voucher for free lead-safety training for a family member. The pre-existing educational materials were provided as bilingual documents, in English and one other language—Spanish, Khmer, or Vietnamese. On a limited basis, materials were also distributed in Russian, Chinese, and Portuguese.
2. Recruitment of community health centers and agencies that serve pregnant women in the target communities (e.g., WIC, Head Start, etc.) to educate their staffs and clients and distribute information kits; and,
3. Sponsorship of Grand Rounds training (offering CEUs) for physicians and other medical and program staff in the four communities.

This project was supported by a nine-month CDC supplemental grant of $100,000.

Jurisdiction or Target Area: Four high-risk communities in Massachusetts (Lawrence, Fitchburg, Lynn, and Holyoke)

Primary Actor: CLPPP, Massachusetts Dept. of Public Health

Secondary Actor(s): N/A

Staffing utilized: Staffing was routinely about 1.25 FTE, but spiked during busy periods associated with trainings and implementation (e.g., about 5 FTEs for a few days).

Other resources utilized: N/A

Factors essential to implementation: Staff felt that success was dependent on the availability of a full-time project coordinator and—for effective materials distribution and training recruitment channels—on the network of existing contacts in the community. MA CLPPP was able to use existing MOUs with some partners, which expedited administrative processes.

Limitations/challenges/problems encountered: Major challenges were in the areas of deadlines and evaluation. Various administrative factors meant that the program had about seven months to hire staff and complete the project, operating within the constraints of state governmental systems for purchasing. Due to time and realities, the program was limited to a self-reporting evaluation. Logistical constraints, including an interpretation of HIPAA requirements, prevented an evaluation approach involving tracking individual women's names.

Magnitude of Impact/Potential Impact: Approximately 3,500 diaper bags/information kits were distributed in 4 months, with many distributed in high-risk areas; 29 agencies signed Memoranda of Understanding (MOU) and partnered in the project; 138 self-reported evaluation cards were returned from kits; and Grand Rounds attendees gave high evaluation marks.

Potential for replication: Moderate

Contacts for Specific Information

Xanthi Scrimgeour
Health Education Coordinator
413-586-7525 x1122 or 1-800-445-1255
Xanthi.Scrimgeour@state.ma.us

Paul Hunter
Director, MA CLPPP
617-624-5585
paul.hunter@state.ma.us

References for additional information
1. An August 2003 report called "CDC Supplemental Prenatal Grant: Overview and Evaluation" describes the project and its results in detail. The report includes a review conducted with the New England Lead Coordinating Council of similar prenatal lead education activities that had been undertaken in other states.

ILLUSTRATION #2 OF STRATEGY IN PRACTICE

As part of a nine-month project focused on increasing testing rates for lead among pregnant women in Alameda and Fresno counties and prompting early intervention, CA CLPPP developed, disseminated, and field-tested educational materials for at-risk pregnant women. To this end, brochures were developed urging women to get tested, and explaining how lead gets into the body, how it can affect a baby, and how to create a lead-safe environment. County-specific phone numbers were provided so that women could easily seek medical care and information regarding lead and pregnancy. After completion, 25,000 packets of culturally-appropriate outreach materials were distributed to high-risk pregnant women and their families through community programs that also provide services to these populations in the two counties, including WIC, Head Start, MediCal, Black Infant Health, and other agencies. 15,000 postcards with a brief "get tested now" message and county phone numbers were also mailed to specific high-risk areas and addresses based on analyses of county tax assessor and Census data. CA CLPPP also conducted direct outreach to medical providers, sponsoring training meetings, distributing educational information, and offering CME/CEU credits. CA CLPPP also sought to help develop and sustain an infrastructure of primary prevention resources for pregnant women and families, beginning with distribution of referral information.

The larger project was supported by a nine-month CDC supplemental grant of $100,000 focused on preventing lead poisoning in at-risk pregnant women and their offspring. The educational materials were tested with 35 participants in a WIC health information class, who provided feedback via a questionnaire and group discussion. Staff were surprised to learn that, despite having used professional translators to develop their materials, there were still some words that were not understood and some graphics that were not clear to the audience.

Jurisdiction or Target Area: Alameda and Fresno Counties in California

Primary Actor: CLPP Branch of CA Dept. of Health Services

Secondary Actor(s): N/A

Staffing utilized: 2 FTE plus 0.5 in-kind

Other resources utilized: N/A

Factors essential to implementation: Project staff felt that the key ingredient for success was the genuine collaboration and support of the community partners. The WIC clinics were particularly effective partners as they already had ongoing and trusting relationships with the pregnant women, and because they incorporated the lead education into their WIC orientation sessions to reinforce the written information.

Limitations/challenges/problems encountered: None.

Magnitude of Impact/Potential Impact: CA CLPPP has not yet been able to measure the larger outcomes of the project, as they are waiting for access to 2003 vital statistic files with data on how many neonates were tested for lead in the target counties. The program will also look at Occupational Lead Poisoning Prevention Branch records for data on how many women were tested in the target counties.

Potential for replication: High

Contact for Specific Information
Laura Jelliffe Pawlowski, PhD
Research Scientist
CA Department of Health Services
Childhood Lead Poisoning Prevention Branch
510-622-4915
LJelliff@dhs.ca.gov

References for additional information
1. CA DHS has available its June 2003 report provided to CDC at the end of the grant period. The report describes project goals and objectives, and reports on project milestones for a larger project designed to increase testing of at-risk pregnant women and provide appropriate interventions.

INTEGRATE LEAD POISONING PREVENTION EDUCATION INTO PHYSICIAN EDUCATION CURRICULA

DESCRIPTION OF THE STRATEGY

Pediatricians who are knowledgeable about lead safety and healthy homes can provide better health care for children at high risk of toxic exposures, advocate for relevant solutions, and suggest primary prevention tools for parents. A recent study revealed that many pediatricians want to better understand lead exposure and other environmental history components in patients' backgrounds, yet fewer than one in five has any formal training in making inquiries on lead and other chemical exposures.

Medical schools and residency review committees can work to train pediatricians in environmental history-taking to identify possible lead exposures in the home and to help prevent exposure. Integrating such specialized training into required medical education is the easiest method, as most medical schools already require some level of lead poisoning prevention education during pediatric clinical rotations. Some state medical societies may get involved in mandating primary prevention education requirements, and residency review committees will also be involved. Requiring a rotation at a children's hospital, community center, or local health department can give pediatric students even more first-hand experience with childhood lead poisoning and add extra incentives for them to take steps toward primary prevention in their future practices. Additional course offerings on primary prevention and environmental history-taking could also be included in physicians' required Continuing Medical Education (CME).

BENEFITS

Immediate/Direct Results: Pediatricians would be formally trained in environmental history-taking and lead hazard inquiry techniques. When interviewing patients, pediatricians would be able to identify potential sources of exposures before at-risk patients become lead poisoned.

Public Health Benefits: Pediatricians would be better able to identify children at risk of lead poisoning, help alert parents to existing lead hazards, and recommend actions to make children's homes lead-safe.

Other Indirect/Collateral Benefits: As pediatricians integrate lead hazard inquiries into routine medical histories, they will help educate parents about lead safety and exposure prevention. Pediatricians are also often trusted, influential members of their communities who could use their knowledge to encourage local, county, and state governments and agencies to expand their use of primary prevention strategies.

SCOPE OF POTENTIAL IMPACT

Statewide   Regional (e.g. multi-county)
City- or County-Wide

PRIMARY ACTORS

Health Department
State Medical Licensing Board
Medical Schools

KEY PARTNERS

State Medical Examinations
State Medical Associations
Certification Boards

CRITICAL ELEMENTS

Staff requirements: No new staff would be required to implement this strategy. A fraction of an FTE would be needed to modify already-existing lead poisoning prevention education to integrate emphasis on primary prevention and environmental history-taking.

Other resource requirements: N/A

Institutional capacity required: Curricula complete with primary prevention and environmental history-taking education is the main institutional requirement for this strategy.

Cost considerations: No additional costs would be incurred if this training on environmental history-taking and lead safety is integrated into existing education and training systems for pediatricians.

Timing issues: None

Feasibility of Implementation: Very high. Because some lead poisoning prevention is already built into most medical school curricula as all students go through their pediatric rotations, putting more emphasis on primary prevention and environmental history-taking would require only modest adjustments to curricula, with little or no conflict with other course priorities.

POTENTIAL OBSTACLES/BARRIERS
None identified.

ADDITIONAL RESOURCES

1. Kilpatrick, et. al., "The Environmental History in Pediatric Practice: A Study of Pediatricians Attitudes, Beliefs, and Practices," *Environmental Health Perspectives*, Vol. 110, No. 8, 823-827, August 2002 http://ehpnet1.niehs.nih.gov/members/2002/110p823-827kilpatrick/kilpatrick-full.html or http://ehpnet1.niehs.nih.gov/members/2002/110p823-827kilpatrick/EHP110p823PDF.PDF

Contacts for Specific Information

Dr. Myrtis Sullivan
Pediatrician and Professor of Environmental Health
Univ. of Illinois-Chicago
312-996-7684
myrtis@uic.edu

Prof. Benjamin Gitterman
Associate Professor of Pediatrics
Children's National Medical Center
George Washington University
202-994-1166
bgitterm@cnmc.org

References for additional information
N/A

ORGANIZE "TOXIC TOURS" FOR POLICY MAKERS

DESCRIPTION OF THE STRATEGY

A first-hand look at unhealthy housing conditions can be provided to public officials by organizing a community tour that allows them to visit homes with hazards (and if possible, some that have been repaired) and talk with residents and advocates about the problems and policy solutions. Experience has shown that policy makers can be moved significantly by the personal experience of seeing hazardous conditions first-hand and having face-to-face interaction with families directly affected. First-year medical students can also benefit from a "toxic tour."

Community-based organizations in Los Angeles, New Orleans, and Providence have successfully used this strategy to educate and motivate local health and housing officials. This strategy parallels "Child Watch" tours that child advocacy groups have historically conducted to sensitize and challenge elected officials and journalists regarding a variety of problems that children face.

BENEFITS

Immediate/Direct Results: As a result of seeing first-hand serious lead hazards and families' otherwise difficult living conditions, government officials are encouraged to step up their response to the problem by improving services to families and fully implementing existing policies.

Public Health Benefits: Tours that include reporters and photojournalists can generate press coverage that builds public understanding of the problem and support for action and policy change.

Other Indirect/Collateral Benefits: Families whose homes are included in the tour have the opportunity to fully explain and show the circumstances they confront. They often feel acknowledged and empowered by the attention of the officials and the media.

SCOPE OF POTENTIAL IMPACT

City- or County-Wide

PRIMARY ACTORS

Community-based Organizations
Tenants

KEY PARTNERS

Health Department
Local Elected Officials

CRITICAL ELEMENTS

Staff requirements: Coordinating a tour can take up to six weeks of full time effort. In addition, all the organizations/agencies involved in the tour need to motivate and mobilize turn-out. It takes ideally 3 people to staff the tour itself: one to serve as navigator, one to confirm with residents in advance of each stop, and one to "emcee" the tour—providing background and context in advance of each location and to reinforce key points and facilitate discussion following each location.

Other resource requirements: N/A

Institutional capacity required: Trusting relationships between the community-based organization and tenants are critical. Tenants are otherwise often afraid to open their homes, fearing retaliation from landlords or criticism and judgment from government officials.

Cost considerations: Transportation for the tour

Timing issues: A tour will be most effective if timed to maximize participation (to coincide with other events, such as a conference) and/or to highlight issues on which decisions are pending (such as budget votes or proposed regulation or legislation), or in advance of local elections.

Feasibility of Implementation: High feasibility.

POTENTIAL OBSTACLES/BARRIERS

It can be quite challenging to convince public officials, especially elected officials, and the media to participate in the tour. Another challenge is ensuring sensitivity to the families who agree to open their homes to the tour. It is a fine line between showcasing the problem and potential solutions vs. unintentionally allowing voyeurism at the expense of low-income families.

ADDITIONAL RESOURCES
N/A

ILLUSTRATION OF STRATEGY IN PRACTICE

The Los Angeles Healthy Homes Collaborative has found that providing public officials with tours of hazardous housing conditions deepens the understanding and motivation to enforce standards and improve services to affected families.

The Healthy Homes Collaborative is a diverse coalition of community-based and advocacy organizations committed to eliminating environmental health threats to children and increasing health access. The Collaborative enlists families whose homes will be visited, persuades agency and legislative staff to attend, and arranges the itinerary, transportation, and food for the attendees. An opportunity for the group to eat together is important to all allow attendees to exchange impressions, information, and ideas.

Jurisdiction or Target Area: Los Angeles, California

Primary Actor: Los Angeles Healthy Homes Collaborative

Secondary Actor(s): N/A

Staffing utilized: 1 FTE

Other resources utilized: N/A

Factors essential to implementation: Because the Collaborative has worked consistently with tenants and earned their trust, the CBO leaders are able to persuade tenants to participate.

Limitations/challenges/problems encountered: The logistics of the tour can be challenging. The size of Los Angeles meant that public officials had to commit almost a full day, with the result that elected officials sent their aides instead of seeing the housing conditions first hand. There may be last-minute conflicts that affect a family's ability to be home or disruptions in the tour schedule, so it is advisable to line up 'extra' families who are willing to participate. Another challenge is facilitating the discussion and reactions of participants with diverse political views and perspectives as everyone is in "close quarters" for the tour.

Magnitude of Impact/Potential Impact: Agency staff felt a new sense of urgency from seeing the desperate living conditions of many families and from seeing how hazards persist in units where violations had been cited. Staff of the lead poisoning prevention program have since been more responsive when alerted to families in need by the Collaborative; communication and working relationships between the CBOs and the agencies have improved.

Potential for replication: High. There is little that prevents community-based organizations or lead poisoning prevention programs across the country from replicating this strategy; indeed it has been effectively implemented by communities to build awareness and public support on a wide range of neighborhood concerns.

Contact for Specific Information

Linda Kite

Coordinator, Los Angeles Healthy Homes Collaborative

213-386-4901

lkite@psr.org

References for additional information

N/A

PUBLICIZE PROBLEM RENTAL PROPERTY OWNERS

DESCRIPTION OF THE STRATEGY

Communities can improve local housing conditions and advance lead poisoning prevention and healthy homes by publicizing "problem landlords" in local media. Publicly drawing attention to repeat violators works to hold property owners accountable, facilitate prosecution of offenders, and deter future offenders. Simultaneously, this strategy increases awareness of the dangers of code violations, builds public and political support for code enforcement, and creates a common cause through which citizens and elected officials can work together.

BENEFITS

Immediate/Direct Results: Owners of substandard housing may be embarrassed by public exposure. Such publicity may serve as deterrence to other landlords, reinforcing the need for improved maintenance. Code inspectors may be empowered and political will increased for stronger enforcement.

Public Health Benefits: As pressure mounts for owners to fix up their properties and repair lead hazards, occupants' risk of exposure to lead will be reduced. Code violations that can lead to other health and housing problems (e.g. mold, rodents, and cockroaches) may be addressed as landlords seek to restore their reputation and public image. In the meantime, potential tenants will avoid these properties and protect their children from risk of exposure.

Other Indirect/Collateral Benefits: Landlords who have not taken code enforcement seriously may be convinced to be more vigilant in addressing problems and performing preventive maintenance. Current tenants in those dwellings may receive assistance not forthcoming prior to the public release of code violation information. Potential tenants will be warned away from properties owned by persons and entities with an established record for code violations including lead-based paint hazards.

SCOPE OF POTENTIAL IMPACT

City- or County-Wide   Neighborhood/Community

PRIMARY ACTORS

Health Department
Code or Building Inspection Agency
Housing Agency
Mayors' Offices

KEY PARTNERS

Tenants
Media

CRITICAL ELEMENTS

Staff requirements: This strategy can be implemented using existing staff.

Other resource requirements: Accurate code violation data, updated on a regular basis, is a key resource.

Institutional capacity required: No special institutional capacity will be required to implement this strategy.

Cost considerations: No added costs will be required for this strategy.

Timing issues: This strategy can be implemented at any time and should be easy to sustain

Feasibility of Implementation: High. This strategy should be relatively easy to implement.

POTENTIAL OBSTACLES/BARRIERS

Some local real estate groups or rental property owners' associations will attempt to discourage elected officials from publishing information that exposes problem landlords.

ADDITIONAL RESOURCES
N/A

ILLUSTRATION OF STRATEGY IN PRACTICE

In September 2003, Indianapolis' mayor unveiled a "Top 10" list of city property owners who have been serial code violators. The property owners on the initial list held title to 310 properties throughout the city. The mayor's list, which is updated as needed, serves several purposes. It helps to distribute information on problem landlords, assisting tenants in avoiding structures that may contain dangerous code violations and health hazards while exposing slumlords to the local community. It also helps the city to hold property owners accountable and provides a tool for community leaders seeking to put pressure on property owners to remedy code violations and maintain their properties.

The list is readily available through the city's website, and it has also been publicized by *The Indianapolis Star* newspaper.

Jurisdiction or Target Area: Indianapolis, Indiana

Primary Actor: The Office of the Mayor

Secondary Actor(s): N/A

Staffing utilized: Less than one week of existing staff's time was needed to compile the list.

Other resources utilized: *The Indianapolis Star* newspaper.

Factors essential to implementation: The willingness of the Mayor's Office to take on problem landlords, as well as the cooperation of *The Indianapolis Star* in publicizing the Top Ten list, have been essential to the implementation of this strategy.

Limitations/challenges/problems encountered: The main challenge in implementing this strategy was compiling information from city and county code inspectors to provide a comprehensive picture of the most serious serial code violators.

Magnitude of Impact/Potential Impact: The Top Ten problem landlords list reached 270,000 *Indianapolis Star* subscribers. The list continues to reach countless others through the city's website.

Potential for replication: The potential for replication is very high.

Contact for Specific Information
Bruce Baird
Administrator of Neighborhood Services Division, Department of Metropolitan Development
317-327-5617
bbaird@indygov.org

References for additional information
1. Mayor Bart Peterson's Top 10 list of problem property owners
    www.indygov.org/eGov/Mayor/home.htm

PUBLICIZE RESTRICTIONS
ON UNSAFE REMODELING AND RENOVATION

DESCRIPTION OF THE STRATEGY

Several cities and states have laws that prohibit renovation and remodeling practices that generate lead dust. Typically, these rules are not enforced, except when officials receive tips about violations from informed and alert individuals. However, the existence of such legal restrictions provides an opportunity to educate the public about the dangers of common paint removal practices, such as uncontained power sanding. Greater awareness can increase the volume of complaints about violations and empower tenants to insist on lead-safe work practices when repairs are done. More widespread knowledge of prohibited practices can also encourage modification of routine work practices to eliminate unsafe methods and prevent the creation of hazards.

BENEFITS

Immediate/Direct Results: Greater awareness can prompt stricter enforcement of laws banning unsafe practices. It can also inform people about ways to prevent inadvertent creation of lead hazards.

Public Health Benefits: As safer work practices are used in the repair or removal of lead-based paint, lead hazards will be avoided and the risks to children will decrease.

Other Indirect/Collateral Benefits: Community-based organizations that build awareness of safe work practice requirements may encourage responsible government agencies to step up their enforcement against unsafe work practices. Partnerships between nonprofit organizations and agencies can put noticeable pressure on contractors and landlords to more widely adopt lead-safe work practices.

SCOPE OF POTENTIAL IMPACT

Statewide

City- or County-Wide

Regional (e.g. multi-county)

Neighborhood/Community

PRIMARY ACTORS

Code or Building Inspection Agency

Community-based Organizations

KEY PARTNERS

Housing Agency

Retail Stores

CRITICAL ELEMENTS

Staff requirements: The production of outreach materials for this strategy may initially require limited staff support.

Other resource requirements: A thorough understanding of federal, state, and local laws governing unsafe work practices is essential.

Institutional capacity required: If publicity is undertaken by a government agency, they may need some regulatory authority underlying their efforts, though this is not always the case.

Cost considerations: Production of simple materials would likely be cost-effective. Distribution costs can be kept down by sending out notices with other government mailings (e.g. tax bills) or engaging the help of businesses to post notices at hardware stores or mail with utility bills.

Timing issues: Timing publicity efforts with other agencies, private companies, or other organizations could lower costs and improve the impact.

Feasibility of Implementation: Very high. This strategy is easily implemented.

POTENTIAL OBSTACLES/BARRIERS

A lack of resources may be the largest potential obstacle for this strategy, as publicizing unsafe work practices will require informational materials and staff time. A lack of cooperation from local agencies, private businesses, or organizations could also be a barrier to successful implementation of this strategy.

ADDITIONAL RESOURCES

N/A

ILLUSTRATION OF STRATEGY IN PRACTICE

In October 2003, IKE and the Lead-Safe Indiana Task Force published pamphlets on lead-based paint hazards. Three pamphlets illustrate practices that are permitted and practices that are banned when working on surfaces that have lead-based paint in Indiana. Two four-page pamphlets are designed for property owners and contractors. The third pamphlet is a two-page document that is sized and designed to be distributed with every issued building permit; it folds to pocket-size so that it can be carried at work sites by contractors and do-it-yourself renovators. The work was funded by a small grant from EPA and the Indiana Department of Environmental Management via the Wayne County Health Department. The documents have been mass-produced and are published on the web for easy downloading and printing.

Jurisdiction or Target Area: Indiana

Primary Actor: Improving Kids' Environment (IKE) and the Lead-Safe Indiana Task Force

Secondary Actor(s): Wayne County Health Dept., Indiana Dept. of Environmental Management, local building inspection agencies

Staffing utilized: 1.5 FTE for a time-limited period.

Other resources utilized: Expertise in lead-safe work practices and Indiana's unsafe work practices law.

Factors essential to implementation: Essential factors included a cooperative working relationship with the Wayne County Health Department; cooperation and information-sharing with the Indiana Department of Environmental Management; and the willingness of local government agencies to participate in publicizing lead-safe work practices information.

Limitations/challenges/problems encountered: No significant challenges or problems have been encountered in IKE's implementation of this strategy.

Magnitude of Impact/Potential Impact: The pamphlets, still relatively new, have already had substantial impact. The web versions of the pamphlets have been downloaded more than 600 times since November 2003. Four local jurisdictions send the pamphlets out with every issued building permit. One Indianapolis property owner that controls roughly 4,500 units mandates that its contractors use the pamphlets in any work with lead-based paint. Anecdotal evidence shows that the pamphlets have made it easier for contractors and property owners to avoid unsafe work practices, and that lead-safe work practices are being more widely adopted.

Potential for replication: The potential for replication is high, especially if a community-based organization has some expertise in lead-safe work practices requirements, as well as good working relationships with other organizations, local government agencies, property owners, and contractors in the region.

Contacts for Specific Information

Tom Neltner
President, Improving Kids' Environment
317-442-3973
neltner@ikecoalition.org

Indiana Dept. of Environmental Management Lead Hotline
1-888-574-8150

References for additional information

1. "Reducing Lead Hazards During Maintenance, Renovation and Abatement," Improving Kids' Environment
   www.ikecoalition.org/documents/Contractor.pdf

2. "Property Managers Responsibilities for Lead-Based Paint," Improving Kids' Environment
   www.ikecoalition.org/documents/PropertyManager.pdf

3. "Now that you have your building permit . . . You must deal with lead-based paint for kids' sake!" Improving Kids' Environment
   www.ikecoalition.org/documents/BuildingPermit.pdf

USE DATA FROM COMMUNITY HOME HAZARD INVESTIGATIONS TO ADVOCATE FOR POLICY SOLUTIONS

DESCRIPTION OF THE STRATEGY

Community organizations can document deteriorated paint, lead dust, and other health hazards in homes using low-tech tools such as those developed by the Community Environmental Health Resource Center (CEHRC) and use the aggregate hazard data to press landlords and government agencies to address hazards in specific properties and to advocate for community-wide solutions.

BENEFITS

Immediate/Direct Results: Using the hazard investigation data, community-based organizations (CBOs) and others can work to win additional resources for hazard remediation, medical attention, and education targeted to communities proven to be at high risk for health hazards in housing. Also, housing not normally tested for hazards under current systems is referred to lead hazard control programs and code agencies responsible for ensuring good housing maintenance and repair.

Public Health Benefits: Residents are encouraged by CBOs and volunteers to have their children tested for lead and are introduced to community resources such as medical clinics, home-buying assistance, and educational opportunities through work with CBOs and other residents. A community-wide picture of lead hazards in housing will help health departments and others to target attention and resources. Media coverage resulting from the release of the data highlights dangers to a wider audience, increasing attention to housing-related health hazards and issues concerning communities at risk in general.

Other Indirect/Collateral Benefits: Community leadership and capacity are built from a greater sense of community among affected residents as they become organized to demand action to address housing-based health hazards as well as other community-wide ills such as ambient pollution and public safety.

SCOPE OF POTENTIAL IMPACT

Statewide   Regional (e.g. multi-county)
City- or County-Wide   Neighborhood/Community

PRIMARY ACTORS

Health Department
Code or Building Inspection Agency
Community-based organizations

KEY PARTNERS

Tenants
Elected Officials

CRITICAL ELEMENTS

Staff requirements: A minimum of 1 FTE capable of managing follow-up with residents whose homes have been found to have hazards (to determine corrective action taken and provide general support to the families) and coordinate and implement an advocacy campaign using data. CBO staff should be able to analyze local policy elements and advocate for new policies or enforcement of existing policies to improve hazard prevention and control at the community-level and beyond. The training of local leaders living in dangerous housing is also a very important staffing element, as these affected local leaders will be the most effective spokespeople on the issue. The initial environmental sampling/data collection phase requires a different staffing pattern, including a cadre of stipendiary community-based volunteers or interns, for example, high school students or VISTA volunteers. These individuals are trained in all of the aspects of environmental sampling and in inviting families to have their homes checked for hazards through door-knocking and making presentations at churches, local health fairs, and block parties.

Other resource requirements: Technical assistance from public agencies; non-profit intermediaries (like the Alliance for Healthy Homes); access to Legal Aid and mapping/GIS technology and skills; media advocacy knowledge/experience; advocacy experience.

Institutional capacity required: Ability to manage a complex program with strict documentation requirements, quality assurance/quality control needs, policy advocacy elements.

Cost considerations: Lead hazard testing lab and material costs are in the range of $60/unit. A meaningful project, covering stipends for hazard investigators and salary for project manager, costs at least $75,000 annually.

Timing issues: None.

Feasibility of Implementation: High. This strategy is feasible for community-based organizations with strong ties to at-risk communities and staff with skills to manage a multifaceted project. Reaching advocacy goals can take many months.

POTENTIAL OBSTACLES/BARRIERS

Actual and perceived state restrictions on who may take lead hazard samples can delay start-up and harm project credibility. Socio-economic factors inherent to the community, including working with potentially vulnerable residents like undocumented immigrants, many of whom are likely to be living in substandard housing. Lack of political will may impede progress on advocacy goals.

ADDITIONAL RESOURCES

1. Community Environmental Health Resource Center
   www.cehrc.org

ILLUSTRATION OF STRATEGY IN PRACTICE

Forty-three percent of New York City's lead poisoned children reside in Brooklyn and the highest concentration of lead poisoned children live in the neighborhoods of Bedford-Stuyvesant and Bushwick. Armed with this knowledge, PACC and Benjamin Banneker secondary school organizers undertook an environmental sampling campaign to prove that the housing in Bedford-Stuyvesant is poisoning low-income residents, and used their results to pressure the city and landlords into protecting these residents by improving the condition of their housing. PACC organizers visited all 200 apartment buildings within a 12-block target area and recruited families to have their units checked for lead hazards. Lead sampling and visual assessment conducted by trained PACC organizers and Banneker students documented lead hazards in 37 percent of the buildings and 32 percent of the individual apartments checked, and the fact that 89 percent of the apartments with hazards housed families with children under age six.

Using this data and other neighborhood demographic information, PACC issued a report on their findings during legislative hearings on a new city lead law and received wide press coverage on television, on radio, and in daily and community newspapers. The report identified several policy failures that PACC found to contribute to the high rate of lead poisoning in this community and offered solutions for corrective action. In general, PACC's findings supported the need for specific remedies, including targeting highest-risk neighborhoods for primary prevention. The report specifically noted that under existing law, there was no mandate for proactive inspections in high-risk areas or requirements for dust testing to prevent poisonings.

Jurisdiction or Target Area: Bedford-Stuyvesant, Fort Greene, Clinton Hill areas of Brooklyn, NY

Primary Actor: Pratt Area Community Council (PACC)

USE DATA FROM COMMUNITY HOME HAZARD INVESTIGATIONS TO ADVOCATE FOR POLICY SOLUTIONS

Secondary Actor(s): N/A

Staffing utilized: 1 FTE, support from various other staff.

Other resources utilized: Lead sampling supplies needed for data collection phase of the project.

Factors essential to implementation: Strong relationships with local churches with undocumented members was an important means to reaching families. The church is one of the only institutions where undocumented immigrants feel relatively safe and able to discuss their housing and other social problems without worrying about political backlash.

Limitations/challenges/problems encountered: Hostility from the City's Departments of Housing Preservation and Development and Health and Mental Hygiene, largely in reaction to negative press generated from study.

Magnitude of Impact/Potential Impact: This campaign highlighted the prevalence of lead hazards in rental properties in this high-risk neighborhood. The substantial media coverage that resulted raised awareness citywide. The campaign triggered repairs in nine of nineteen dangerous units discovered; produced a report that was cited in City Council hearings; and provided a model for other organizations.

Potential for replication: High. This strategy is replicable given funding for data and political analysis, staff, and technical assistance.

Contact for Specific Information
Gabriel Thompson
Lead Organizer, PACC
718-522-2613
Gabriel_Thompson@prattarea.org

References for additional information
1. "The Politics of Poison", Pratt Area Community Council. Amy Laura Cahn and Gabriel Thompson. (2003)
   www.nmic.org/nyccelp/documents/PACC-Report.pdf
2. Tenant/Inquilino newsletter, Metropolitan Council on Housing, New York, NY, Summer 2003.
   www.tenant.net/Tengroup/Metcounc/Jul03/jul03.pdf
3. "1 in 3 Children in Brooklyn Area Exposed to Dangerous Lead Levels, a Study Finds," *New York Times*, June 9, 2003.
4. "The Politics of Paint," *City Limits*, September/October 2003.
   www.citylimits.org

USE INVESTIGATIVE JOURNALISM TO REVEAL DIMENSIONS OF THE PROBLEM AND POLICY SHORTCOMINGS

DESCRIPTION OF THE STRATEGY

Effective journalism builds public support for solutions by "putting a human face on the problem." Community-based organizations can increase awareness and promote needed policy solutions by guiding investigative reporters to stories that reveal the hidden dimensions of healthy housing problems and the shortcomings of existing programs and systems, and government agency staff can respond to media inquiries with official data and information on current policies. Examples of powerful investigative series that galvanized support for lead poisoning prevention are Jim Haner's 2000 series in the *Baltimore Sun,* Peter Lord's May 2002 series in the *Providence Journal,* the 2003 series and continuing coverage by a team of reporters at the Detroit *Free Press,* and Luis Perez' continuing coverage in the Syracuse newspapers.

BENEFITS

Immediate/Direct Results: The immediate result is an increase in public attention to and understanding of the problem. Groundbreaking reporting often generates coverage by other media, further building public awareness.

Public Health Benefits: Heightened awareness frequently translates in increased political support for policy change. In particular, elected officials feel considerable pressure to respond to the problem and demonstrate that they are making improvements. Elected officials are more amenable to new policy proposals and and/or to deciding on pending proposals and breaking long-standing deadlocks over policy solutions.

Other Indirect/Collateral Benefits: Very often the families featured in coverage of lead poisoning feel acknowledged, validated, and empowered by the coverage. The reporting is often the first time that they see their problems and struggles taken seriously, and that their situation can help contribute to solving the problem for other families.

SCOPE OF POTENTIAL IMPACT

Statewide   Regional (e.g. multi-county)
City- or County-Wide   Neighborhood/Community
Specific (Targeted) Population—Elected Officials

PRIMARY ACTORS

Newspapers

KEY PARTNERS

Health Department
Housing Agency
Community-based Organizations
Tenants
General Public

CRITICAL ELEMENTS

Staff requirements: This strategy can be implemented by existing staff. Prompting effective media coverage requires a willingness to reach out to the press and to invest time and effort into helping them understand all the aspects of health hazards in the home environment. Because most reporters are generalists and will likely be new to the subject, CBOs and advocates need to be patient and persistent in helping the reporter master the topic and find ways to present it to the public that will foster new understanding. While some may be reluctant to trust reporters, openness and cooperation create opportunities to shape the coverage. Persistent outreach to reporters can educate them about the issue and raise its profile to the extent that it becomes one that news organizations can't ignore and will invest considerable resources in covering.

Other resource requirements: Official data can help ground the coverage in facts and illuminate the problem in compelling ways. Electronic copies of address-based data are especially useful to getting graphic displays, such as maps, published. Digital photographs of hazardous conditions, code violations, and repair work can facilitate press coverage and add punch to stories.

Institutional capacity required: N/A

Cost considerations: Extremely low cost.

Timing issues: Sustained cultivation of or accessibility to the media is critical; one-time or occasional efforts will be much less effective.

Feasibility of Implementation: Very high

POTENTIAL OBSTACLES/BARRIERS

A potential barrier is the reluctance of families to participate because they fear retaliation from the landlord or other consequences. The willingness of families to cooperate with reporters is essential because the personal toll of lead poisoning helps capture the public attention and build political will to change the status quo.

ADDITIONAL RESOURCES

N/A

ILLUSTRATION #1 OF STRATEGY IN PRACTICE

In May of 2001, the *Providence Journal* ran a six-part series on lead poisoning that helped set the stage for new legislation and regulations in the state. A photojournalist at the *Journal*, John Freidah initiated the idea, but it could not have happened without the commitment of the newspaper, the hard work of the Childhood Lead Action Project, the time and effort of many government officials who educated and provided information to reporter Peter Lord, and the willingness of many families to open their lives to the journalists and the public.

Jurisdiction or Target Area: Rhode Island

Primary Actor: *Providence Journal*

Secondary Actor(s): Childhood Lead Action Project; Rhode Island Department of Health; Rhode Island Housing and Mortgage Finance Corporation

Staffing utilized: At the *Journal*, reporter Peter Lord and photojournalist John Freidah invested more than 6 months of time preparing the series (and Freidah had begun taking photographs at the lead clinic many months earlier in between other assignments in order to bring the idea vividly to the paper's editors). Top editors at the paper worked with them on "designing" the series to most effectively convey the breadth and impact of lead poisoning in the state. At the Childhood Lead Action Project, a community organizer working with the parents of lead-poisoned children helped the parents overcome their fear of participating in the series. Officials at the Rhode Island Department of Health and the Rhode Island Housing and Mortgage Finance Corporation devoted many meetings to helping Peter Lord understand and accurately convey the issues.

Other resources utilized: The state health department forged a partnership with the *Providence Journal* to make public information about properties that have lead hazards. The department had generated a list of houses where children had been poisoned but didn't have the technical capacity to publish it online. By providing these data to the newspaper and by providing yearly updates to the paper, the department has met the public need for information despite its technical limitations.

Factors essential to implementation: The most important factor is that the local newspaper has a commitment to journalism in the public interest and the capacity to commit resources to investigate the issue in depth and devote significant space to telling the story. Equally important is a local community-based organization that can help the reporter dig into the story, intercede to encourage families to participate, and take advantage of the heightened visibility to promote policy change.

Limitations/challenges/problems encountered: None.

Magnitude of Impact/Potential Impact: Within a month after the series, the Rhode Island Department of Health agreed that persistent elevated blood levels of 15-19 would become the threshold for intervention. Advocates, who had long sought the change (from a single EBL of 20 µg/dL), conducted a demonstration at the Department of Health during the week the series appeared, and attribute the change to the heightened awareness combined with timely advocacy action. Within a year after the series, the Rhode Island legislature passed new legislation to hold landlords accountable if a child is poisoned by lead hazards in their properties. Both the bill's sponsor, Senator Thomas Izzo, and the Governor credited the *Journal* series with breaking the deadlock on legislation that had been debated for many years. Every legislator had a copy of the series, which brought home the severity of the problem and made the scope and impact impossible for them to ignore.

Potential for replication: Very high

Contacts for Specific Information

Peter Lord
Reporter, *Providence Journal*
401-227-8036
plord@projo.com

Roberta Aaronson
Director, Childhood Lead Action Project
401-785-1310
executivedirector@leadsafekids.org

References for additional information
1. *Poisoned: Public Health Crisis* by Peter Lord and John Freidah, May 13-18, 2001 *Providence Journal.*

ILLUSTRATION #2 OF STRATEGY IN PRACTICE

The Detroit *Free Press* conducted an in-depth investigation of lead poisoning in Detroit and Michigan that began appearing January 21, 2003. The paper followed the five-day investigative series with continuing coverage throughout the year. The reporting—and the persistent work of state advocates for children's environmental health—resulted in lead poisoning becoming a top priority of the Governor and the state legislature. In addition, the series prompted the US EPA to order the removal of lead-contaminated soil in a Detroit neighborhood near a former lead smelter.

Jurisdiction or Target Area: Michigan

Primary Actor: Detroit *Free Press*

Secondary Actor(s): Get The Lead Out Coalition

Staffing utilized: The *Free Press* devoted a multi-talented team of reporters to covering this issue over many months. The reporters worked with and wrote about families affected by lead poisoning, investigated and identified systemic shortcomings in the city and state's programs, hired experts to test the soil near industrial sites, and researched how local efforts compared with other cities and states around the country. When state advocates, including the Get The Lead Out coalition in Grand Rapids, became aware of the investigation, they provided information to the reporters about the extent of the problem outside Detroit and the need for statewide leadership on lead poisoning prevention. Both the newspaper and the advocates worked to sustain the impact of the initial investigation by continued coverage of the problem and of the policy initiatives of the Governor and the state legislature.

Other resources utilized: The *Free Press* conducted an analysis of the State Department of Community Health data on elevated blood lead levels to identify the "hot spot" neighborhoods—those with the most lead-poisoned children—and questioned why the state had not been using the data to target prevention and hazard control efforts. The analysis revealed that the single worst hot spot was in Grand Rapids—a finding that changed the political dynamic of the issue within the state by capturing the attention of the legislators in the western part of the state, educating them on the scope of the problem statewide, and motivating them to support new legislation. Because the paper had to sue the state to release the data, this article appeared in July, putting the issue back on the front burner six months after the original series.

Factors essential to implementation: The critical factors are a large-circulation newspaper with a commitment to doing investigative reporting, strong advocates who can use the heightened public attention and concern to build political will for policy change, and continuing coverage and advocacy to keep elected officials focused on and accountable for making necessary changes.

Limitations/challenges/problems encountered: The main policy-making challenge in Michigan was overcoming the east/west split in the state. The *Free Press* broadened their focus beyond Detroit and the eastern part of the state at the urging of state advocates. Most legislators had considered lead poisoning a Detroit problem until the *Free Press* analysis of the data documented the extent of the problem in Grand Rapids and other western areas.

Magnitude of Impact/Potential Impact: While the Governor had campaigned as a champion of children's environmental health, it is clear that the investigative series combined with advocates' work to take maximal advantage of the publicity persuaded the Governor to submit a much stronger action plan much more quickly than would otherwise have been the case. It is likely the legislature would have reacted far more coolly to the Governor's proposals without the series. (The bills currently working their way through Michigan House and Senate would establish a Childhood Lead Poisoning Prevention and Control Commission, impose penalties on landlords who knowingly rent units with lead hazards, provide tax credits for lead hazard control, create a lead-safe housing registry, increase pressure on Medicaid plans to screen enrolled children for lead poisoning, and require labs to report blood screening results electronically.)

Potential for replication: High

Contacts for Specific Information

Emilia Askari
Reporter, Detroit *Free Press*
313-223-4461
askari@freepress.com

Paul Haan
Director, Get The Lead Out Coalition
616-241-3300
gtlo@sbcglobal.net

References for additional information

1. *Damaged Lives: Lead's Toxic Toll* January 21-25, 2003, Detroit *Free Press*; and continuing coverage
    www.freep.com/lead/index.htm

BUILDING CAPACITY FOR LEAD SAFETY

ADD LEAD SAFETY TO WEATHERIZATION PROGRAMS AND PRACTICES

ASSESS AND ADDRESS MULTIPLE HAZARDS SIMULTANEOUSLY

BROADCAST LEAD SAFETY TRAINING WIDELY

ENSURE THAT DO-IT-YOURSELF REHABBERS ARE TRAINED

EQUIP COMMUNITY-BASED ORGANIZATIONS AND SERVICE PROVIDERS

EQUIP DAY LABORERS TO WORK SAFELY

EXPAND WEATHERIZATION AND REHAB PROGRAMS TO ADDRESS LEAD SAFETY

HOLD REGULAR LEAD-SAFE WORK PRACTICE TRAININGS

PROVIDE TECHNICAL ASSISTANCE TO PROPERTY OWNERS

TRAIN AND EMPLOY LOW-INCOME COMMUNITY RESIDENTS IN HAZARD CONTROL

ADD LEAD SAFETY TRAINING TO WEATHERIZATION PROGRAMS AND PRACTICES

DESCRIPTION OF THE STRATEGY

Integrating lead safety into the ongoing work of weatherization program contractors has the multiple benefits of reducing energy costs, improving the indoor climate, reducing lead hazards in the homes treated by the weatherization program, improving the safety of weatherization crew workers and their families, and protecting the safety of residents. Lead poisoning prevention programs can provide training and incentives such as free or discounted HEPA vacuums and personal protective equipment. Options include developing a hybrid training curriculum, adding lead-safe work practices to standards or specifications, expanding monitoring and inspections to address lead safety concerns, offering complete lead-safe work practices (LSWP) training within the weatherization training program, subsidizing risk assessor training, and providing an XRF analyzer for each local weatherization program.

BENEFITS

The Department of Energy requires its state-level grantees to ensure that weatherization crews complete lead safety training if they will be working on homes built before 1978. This federal requirement prevents any confusion surrounding the need for lead safety training and ensures that all weatherization workers who operate in older homes will understand the consequences of repair and energy measures that may cut, sand, or pry lead-based paint and how to avoid creating lead dust and paint hazards through proper containment, control during the work, and clean up. It is most efficient to have the state weatherization agency condition disbursement of federal weatherization funds on fulfilling the training requirement; the state can also incorporate into standard training any state-specific standards or other information.

Immediate/Direct Results: There will be increased awareness of lead safety among thousands of laborers and contractors.

Public Health Benefits: Crews will be significantly less likely to create hazards such as lead dust, lead soil, or deteriorated lead paint during weatherization work that disturbs lead-based paint.

Other Indirect/Collateral Benefits: Lead safety capacity is built in the wider community of individuals and community action agencies that may also conduct repair and renovation work using HUD funds or other resources. Transferable lead safety skills will cause laborers who work in weatherization to be careful about paint chips and dust when performing other types of work in older homes in the future. Weatherization program staff gains awareness of potential health risks associated with lead hazards and other housing condition problems. Finally, the initiative helps build capacity among contractors and awareness of lead-safe work practices that will likely transfer to other non-weatherization jobs—when working in older homes likely to have lead based paint.

SCOPE OF POTENTIAL IMPACT

Nationally, the risk of lead dust hazards will be reduced as weatherization crews treat pre-1978 homes. More than 100,000 homes are treated by weatherization each year, and a significant majority were built before 1978.

Statewide—You can pursue such training at the state, county, or local level. It is most efficient to have the state condition disbursement of federal weatherization funds on fulfilling the training requirement.

Regional (e.g. multi-county)—Many CAP agencies cover
City- or County-Wide
Neighborhood/Community
Specific (Targeted) Population—Very low-income households

PRIMARY ACTORS

Weatherization Agencies

KEY PARTNERS

Health Department
Housing Agency
Advocates
Contractors
Workers
Utility companies/agencies
Accredited lead training providers

CRITICAL ELEMENTS

Staff requirements: Developing and implementing lead safety training for weatherization programs can be performed by existing weatherization staff. Existing HUD- and EPA-approved training can be downloaded from the Internet. Ensuring that all workers are trained should be integrated into local staff orientation as well as local and state performance monitoring systems.

Other resource requirements: There are limited resource requirements. The materials that are used in working lead-safely are already part of the typical weatherization toolkit. Training is best accomplished with some hands-on experiences, including visits to homes receiving weatherization treatment where the work is disturbing lead-based paint.

Institutional capacity required: The state weatherization program should fund the training, provide other support, and help trouble-shoot, with assistance from the state's lead poisoning prevention program as needed. States with centralized weatherization training centers should add lead-safe work practices to their existing training program. Other states, as well as local agencies, should equip the trainer(s) who normally provides training to deliver lead safety training so that it is added to the core weatherization curriculum. In some states, this may involve getting accreditation for the trainer. Any class offered in LSWP must be approved by the U.S. Department of Housing and Urban Development; www.hud.gov/offices/lead/training/hudapproval_main.cfm. LIHEAP funds might also be used to subsidize the risk assessor training or purchase XRF machines as a "supply" line item.

Cost considerations: The costs of offering training fluctuate; trainers may charge $600 - $1,600 for a day of training.

Timing issues: An agency or organization can quickly organize training since the courses exist, the requirements are in place from DOE, and no special training facilities are needed. Ongoing training is needed to reach new hires.

Feasibility of Implementation: High. This training is feasible in all state and localities.

POTENTIAL OBSTACLES/BARRIERS

Little or no training will occur without the support of the state weatherization program, which must visibly and vocally support training. The state manager can play a critical role in supporting the effort, issuing clear policy requiring training to occur and providing funding and taking other steps necessary to ensure that the local programs and their staff complete the training.

ADDITIONAL RESOURCES

1. www.waptac.org — A DOE-sponsored site for weatherization programs that describes LSWP training and the existing DOE requirement to complete training.

ILLUSTRATION OF THE STRATEGY IN PRACTICE

This program brings subsidized lead safety training to all agencies administering weatherization funds, provides training to workers, ensures at least one individual is trained and licensed as a lead risk assessor, and provides at least one XRF analyzer to each agency performing weatherization work. The program has developed specific policies and procedures to address lead that are more extensive than the federal requirements. Each weatherization program's risk assessor tests the lead content of the paint likely to be disturbed by the weatherization project in all pre-1978 homes. Using an XRF takes the guesswork out of the job: the crew knows if there is lead paint and does not have to presume it exists. The state pays expert consultants to work with each risk assessor on using the equipment and procedure properly in order to guarantee consistent performance.

Jurisdiction or Target Area: Indiana.

Primary Actor: Division of Family and Children, Housing and Community Service in the Department of Family and Social Services Agency.

Secondary Actor(s): N/A

Staffing utilized: The state weatherization program director helped launch and develop the program with support from one key staffer and an independent consultant. It quickly became a relatively small aspect of the staff person's job as details fell into place. A consultant developed the policies and procedures, and Environmental Management Institute, an accredited lead trainer, was contracted to support the risk assessors.

Other resources utilized: Administrative funding from the Section 8 program was used to purchase XRF devices.

Factors essential to implementation: The key factor for success is the commitment of state weatherization staff who care about the lead issue and are willing to make it a priority. The initial training is relatively easy to get off the ground; maintaining training requires a long-term commitment to integrate lead training into the existing state training of weatherization contractors. In 2003, approximately 100 staff and contractors completed the LSWP course offered by the ongoing weatherization training program. Ongoing funding to continue training is provided by the state weatherization program, which also uses other federal housing and Low Income Heating Energy Assistance Program (LIHEAP) funds to support the effort.

Limitations/challenges/problems encountered: One challenge is to convince key senior managers at the state level of the necessity of creating systems to incorporate lead safety into weatherization and approval for a centralized procurement for XRFs to substantially reduce the price. Obtaining commitments from local community action agency directors to have their weatherization crews complete the training was another challenge that was overcome by the state's upfront provision of needed resources.

Magnitude of Impact/Potential Impact: Weatherization work is performed using lead-safe work practices in all units that have lead-based paint. XRF testing has allowed the CAP agencies to focus dust containment and cleanup efforts when the surface tests positive for lead. Information developed from the lead testing is now available to future tenants and buyers under the federal lead hazard disclosure requirement.

Potential for replication: High. Lead safety training for weatherization crews can be replicated throughout all states in which it is a priority for key managers at the state level.

Contacts for Specific Information

Erica Burrin
Weatherization Specialist
Div of Family and Children
Housing and Community Service, FSSA
317-234-1971
eburrin@fssa.state.in.us

Tom Neltner
President, Improving Kids Environment
317-442-3973
neltner@ikecoalition.org

References for additional information

1. Lead Safe Work Practices Policy for Indiana Weatherization Programs—contact eburrin@fssa.state.in.us
2. Program Flow Chart—contact eburrin@fssa.state.in.us

ASSESS AND ADDRESS MULTIPLE HAZARDS SIMULTANEOUSLY

DESCRIPTION OF THE STRATEGY

Programs that address health hazards beyond lead can efficiently and effectively equip families to reduce health hazards in the home environment. Community-based organizations train community members to assess houses for hazards and leverage the results through both individual and systems advocacy. Such programs also work to build support for prevention through the education of tenants/residents about hazards, available remedies for obtaining safe repairs, legal rights, and leadership skills. Programs focusing on direct services train volunteers and community health workers to conduct home audits, create a personalized Home Action Plan that emphasizes low- or no-cost solutions, and provide tools to assist in making needed changes, such as sealed mattress covers, cleaning kits, and HEPA vacuum loaners.

BENEFITS

Immediate/Direct Results: Home heath hazards will be identified. Rental property owners, their tenants, and owner-occupants will learn low-cost solutions to address hazards and be aware of home health hazards.

Public Health Benefits: Written reports and photographs that are property-specific inform the landlord about hazards. With respect to lead, the landlord then must correct the problem or disclose this information to prospective tenants. Property-specific data transforms the federal lead hazard disclosure rule's right to know into a powerful catalyst for action to improve conditions in substandard rental properties. Aggregate data can motivate local lawmakers to address the prevalence of hazards through property maintenance codes, health and housing codes, and other policy changes.

Other Indirect/Collateral Benefits: Fosters community building and community organizing. Advocates can use aggregate data to generate media interest in the plight of low-income families who seek healthy housing.

SCOPE OF POTENTIAL IMPACT

City- or County-Wide   Neighborhood/ Community

PRIMARY ACTORS	KEY PARTNERS
Community-based Organizations	Rental Property Owners
	Tenants
	General Public and Consumers
	Volunteers

CRITICAL ELEMENTS

Staff requirements: Depending on the type of program implemented, between 1-2 FTE.

Other resource requirements: Standard office equipment, computer equipment, and supplies to check homes for hazards.

Institutional Capacity Required: N/A

Cost considerations: Funding.

Timing issues: Groups may want to begin with the highest risk neighborhoods to generate the most dramatic results.

Feasibility of Implementation: Moderate. Volunteers are the backbone of home assessment programs, which makes them relatively inexpensive to start. However, staffing must be in place to work to retain volunteers and manage their work.

POTENTIAL OBSTACLES/BARRIERS

If home assessments reveal health hazards in rental housing, steps must be taken to ensure that tenants are protected from retaliatory evictions and other illegal landlord actions. Advocates must also guard against the responsibility being inappropriately shifted from landlord to tenant. Advocates must press code inspectors to inspect, cite, and enforce the code.

ADDITIONAL RESOURCES

N/A

ILLUSTRATION #1 OF STRATEGY IN PRACTICE

The American Lung Association of Washington established the Master Home Environmentalist (MHE) program in 1992 and has trained more than 1,400 volunteers. Trainers include environmental scientists, psychologists, social workers, academics, and medical professionals. Volunteers complete 35 hours of training and 35 hours of community service. Trained MHE volunteers use a Home Environmental Assessment List (HEAL™) to help identify health hazards in the home, including lead, dust, and mold. The volunteer then works with the resident to develop an action plan to create a healthier home environment, emphasizing inexpensive or no-cost solutions.

Jurisdiction or Target Area: King County, Washington; expanding to additional counties.

Primary Actor: American Lung Association of Washington

Secondary Actor(s): N/A

Staffing utilized: At a minimum, one full-time staff person is needed to recruit volunteers and members for the steering committee, schedule trainings, etc.

Other resources utilized: Computer, LCD projector for presentations, and trainings are helpful.

Factors essential to implementation: Developing key partners to serve as trainers and on the steering committee is essential. The expertise of key partners depends on the geographical area and the type of classes needed; for example, pesticide experts must be recruited where pesticides are a main issue.

Limitations/challenges/problems encountered: Funding and volunteer retention were both challenges.

Magnitude of Impact/Potential Impact: From 1994 to 1999, MHE volunteers reported completing more than 4,500 hours of community service and 1,400 home assessments. A 1997 study revealed that 86% of households visited by MHE volunteers improved their home environment.

Potential for replication: Moderate. MHE sells its trademarked and licensed program. Purchasers receive the Implementation Guide, training manual, facilitator's guide, HEAL paperwork, database to track volunteers and residents, as well as all components created by other licensees. The cost is $2,500 for an American Lung Association affiliate; the cost is higher for non-affiliates.

Contact for Specific Information
Aileen Gagney
Environmental Health Program Manager
206-441-5100
agagney@alaw.org

References for additional information

1. The American Lung Association of Washington
    www.alaw.org/air_quality/master_home_environmentalist/index.html

ILLUSTRATION #2 OF STRATEGY IN PRACTICE

The Community Environmental Health Resource Center (CEHRC) is a resource for grassroots groups working for social justice in low-income communities around the country. CEHRC provides local organizations with hazard assessment tools and training in their use, technical assistance, strategy advice, and sub-grants. Depending on the hazard, the training may take from 2-3 hours to two days. Community-based organizations undertaking CEHRC projects focus on high-risk rental housing, offer home hazard assessments at no charge, inform residents of the results, and engage and advocate for systems change.

Jurisdiction or Target Area: National

Primary Actor: Community Environmental Health Resource Center (CEHRC), Washington DC

Secondary Actor(s): N/A

Staffing utilized: To implement the CEHRC protocols, a local organization needs 1.5-2.25 FTEs devoted to this project, along with time from shared administrative and support staff.

Other resources utilized: Computer access and funding to provide volunteer stipends are needed. CEHRC provides training in hazard assessment and centralized lab analysis of samples, along with standardized forms and reports, including a resident agreement.

Factors essential to implementation: Community-based organizations must have strong ties to the community, adequate funding, and a strong project manager. Vigorous outreach to target communities is critical to successful projects.

Limitations/challenges/problems encountered: Project management is challenging, as it requires volunteer management, quality control, data collection and upkeep, reporting, inventory maintenance, and other paperwork heavy tasks. Even with a stipend, there may be attrition of volunteers. Residents in high-risk communities may be resistant to letting volunteers in to assess their homes; using volunteers from these areas, especially where language barriers may exist, helped overcome this challenge. In some cases, those testing homes may need to get state-certified.

Magnitude of Impact/Potential Impact: Through the six first-round grantees, more than 1,500 housing units were assessed. CEHRC's tenant/community organizing component has shown success in many project communities, with local groups already generating additional projects.

Potential for replication: Very high. In addition to assistance to its sub-grantees, CEHRC provides technical assistance to community organizations that want to implement home hazard assessment programs. Assistance includes guidance in the mechanics of hazard assessment, prevention, and control and the development of strategies to address these problems. All CEHRC materials are available free on its website; any community-based organization can access them.

Contact for Specific Information
Julia Burgess
CEHRC Director
202-543-1147
jburgess@afhh.org

References for additional information
1. CEHRC
   www.cehrc.org/

BROADCAST LEAD SAFETY TRAINING WIDELY

DESCRIPTION OF THE STRATEGY

Widespread availability and access to training in lead-safe work practices is essential. Using existing public and private telecommunication systems to broadcast training in lead-safe work practices and permit interaction between instructors and class participants can greatly increase the reach of the program. This method of delivery not only conserves travel funds and time but also provides the ability to reach numerous locations and instruct a virtually unlimited number of the broad array of individuals needing the training.

BENEFITS

Immediate/Direct Results: Hundreds, potentially thousands, of landlords, maintenance staff, contractors, laborers, painters, homeowners, and others can be trained in lead-safe work practices at low cost.

Public Health Benefits: As more people are trained in lead-safe work practices, fewer lead hazards will be created during remodeling, renovation, and repair of homes and apartments.

Other Indirect/Collateral Benefits: States will maximize their prior investment in telecommunications technologies (e.g. interactive fiber optics networks). An atmosphere of learning and cooperation can also be fostered among the diverse array of individuals who would benefit from widely broadcast training sessions.

SCOPE OF POTENTIAL IMPACT

Statewide   Regional (e.g. multi-county)

City- or County-Wide   Neighborhood/Community

PRIMARY ACTORS

Code or Building Inspection Agency
Housing Agency
University/county Extension Offices

KEY PARTNERS

Health Department
Community-based Organizations
Property Owners
Contractors
Painters
Homeowners

CRITICAL ELEMENTS

Staff requirements: Staff requirements will vary. For an ongoing program, it is reasonable to assume 0.5 FTE for each trainer, and very limited staff time for set-up of the county or city-based facilities.

Other resource requirements: This strategy requires that a widely accessible, statewide or region-wide telecommunications system be in place. Some states have such systems, accessible on the county level, through university Extension offices, or through other means; other states' systems are more limited. Advertising can also be used to reach the target audience about the training opportunity.

Institutional capacity required: Trainers must be accredited and should be well versed in conducting lead-safe work practices courses.

Cost considerations: This strategy is highly cost-effective. Travel and meal costs will be small or non-existent, and in most areas, needed telecommunications systems already exist and can be used for a modest hourly rate, usually between $12-16 per hour.

Timing issues: This strategy could be implemented at any time.

Feasibility of Implementation: High. In states or regions of states where widespread telecommunication delivery systems exist, this strategy should be feasible. Some limitations may exist.

POTENTIAL OBSTACLES/BARRIERS

There should be few, if any, potential barriers to implementation of this strategy. Hands-on portions of the training will be nearly impossible to conduct using this strategy, which could limit the value of this particular type of lead-safe work practices course.

ADDITIONAL RESOURCES

N/A

ILLUSTRATION OF STRATEGY IN PRACTICE

The Iowa Department of Public Health Bureau of Lead Poisoning Prevention (the Bureau) partnered with the Iowa Department of Economic Development, Iowa's housing agency, public housing authorities, and entitlement cities to produce and deliver a lead-safe work practices training curriculum that could be broadcast to workers who were widely scattered throughout rural and urban Iowa.

Previously, work practices training was delivered through 17 agencies and reached 708 individuals throughout the state of Iowa. HUD had offered a contractor to conduct training for these individuals, but the sessions were limited to two cities, and rural Iowans were unwilling or unable to travel long distances for eight hours worth of training.

To solve this problem, the Bureau decided to utilize the Iowa Communications Network (ICN) to reach hundreds of workers at a time through county facilities. The ICN is a statewide, state-administered, fiber optics network. There are currently over 700 sites in Iowa with connections to the ICN. The ICN utilizes high quality, full-motion video. There is interaction between the originating site and all remote sites, which allowed for full training sessions without the cost or hassle of long-distance travel.

Jurisdiction or Target Area: Iowa

Primary Actor: Iowa Department of Public Health Bureau of Lead Poisoning Prevention

Secondary Actor(s): Iowa Department of Economic Development, Iowa's housing agency, public housing authorities, and entitlement cities.

Staffing utilized: While the training effort was ongoing, 5 FTE were required.

Other resources utilized: The Iowa Communications Network, a fiber optics telecommunications network linked to hundreds of local sites.

Factors essential to implementation: The existence of the ICN was the most important factor to implementing this strategy. However, partnerships with local housing agencies, including public housing authorities and housing rehab offices, were also critical. The local agencies provided a site monitor for each training session, and they also recruited training participants. Funding for this project was provided by the National Center for Healthy Housing to build capacity for implementing HUD's lead-safe housing rule.

Limitations/challenges/problems encountered: The main challenge to implementation was coordination of training materials, Bureau staff, and the training schedule. However, Bureau staff noted that this became easier as time passed.

Magnitude of Impact/Potential Impact: 1,020 landlords and contractors were trained via the ICN.

Potential for replication: High. This strategy can be easily replicated in any state or multi-county region with a fiber optic or other telecommunications presentation and delivery system.

Contact for Specific Information
Rita Gergely
Chief, Bureau of Lead Poisoning Prevention
515-242-6340 or 800-972-2026
rgergely@idph.state.ia.us

References for additional information
N/A

ENSURE THAT DO-IT-YOURSELF REHABBERS ARE TRAINED

DESCRIPTION OF THE STRATEGY

Housing agencies that provide funds for housing rehab can require that property owners be prepared to effectively deal with existing conditions as well as problems that emerge as they work. Rehabbers of older housing especially need to know how to work safely around lead-based paint and how to safely and thoroughly repair lead-based paint hazards. Rehabbers also need to be aware of the U.S. Environmental Protection Agency's Pre-Renovation and Education Program (406b), which requires property owners to notify all occupants in pre-1978 housing units of any rehab work that will disturb more than two square feet of a painted surface.

BENEFITS

Immediate/Direct Results: Training do-it-yourself rehabbers will make it more likely that lead-safe work practices will be used. This will bring a category of properties under the lead-safe work practices umbrella that has been missed through other, more formal training of professional rehabilitation contractors.

Public Health Benefits: Properties that would not otherwise have had the benefit of lead-safe work practices can now be rehabbed safely. This will reduce or eliminate the creation of lead hazards and encourage the repair of existing hazards, which will decrease children's exposure.

Other Indirect/Collateral Benefits: When included as part of a larger housing or development program, this strategy can also help reduce urban blight, reduce other health hazards in older structures, and assist in comprehensive community development and/or revitalization.

SCOPE OF POTENTIAL IMPACT

Statewide

City- or County-Wide

Specific (Targeted) Population

Regional (e.g. multi-county)

Local Community

PRIMARY ACTORS

Housing Agency

KEY PARTNERS

Property Owners

CRITICAL ELEMENTS

Staff requirements: This strategy will require staff time to conduct trainings. This could require up to 1.5 FTE if staff training is provided directly by the funding agency. The agency could also contract with outside trainers.

Other resource requirements: Lead-safe work practices training materials will be necessary for this strategy.

Institutional capacity required: Training instructors should be well versed in lead-safe work practices.

Cost considerations: This strategy should be cost-effective in preventing health problems.

Timing issues: This strategy would require some short-duration outreach, but it can be implemented at any time. It is also important to implement this strategy in a sustainable way so as to not limit its effectiveness.

Feasibility of Implementation: Very high in almost all jurisdictions.

POTENTIAL OBSTACLES/BARRIERS

Few, if any, barriers should exist for this strategy.

ADDITIONAL RESOURCES

N/A

ILLUSTRATION OF STRATEGY IN PRACTICE

The City of Rocky Mount, North Carolina offers free home maintenance and repair classes to area homeowners and rental property owners every year. The two-hour class covers a variety of topics, including lead awareness and lead-safe work practices. Other class topics are also directly or indirectly related to preventing the creation of lead hazards, such as keeping moisture under control by repairing roofing and siding, properly maintaining plumbing fixtures, and utilizing energy conservation measures. The classes are open to the general public and are also required for anyone seeking housing rehab assistance from the city.

Jurisdiction or Target Area: City of Rocky Mount, North Carolina

Primary Actor: Rocky Mount Planning and Development Department

Secondary Actor(s): N/A

Staffing utilized: 0.5 FTE over 4 months each year.

Other resources utilized: N/A

Factors essential to implementation: The most essential factor to the implementation of this strategy was the interest of area residents, homeowners, and rental property owners in the free classes.

Limitations/challenges/problems encountered: No significant challenges or problems were encountered in implementing this strategy.

Magnitude of Impact/Potential Impact: The training classes have reached over 200 people in the Rocky Mount area.

Potential for replication: Very high. Rocky Mount's version of this strategy is low-cost, utilizing existing staff in the Planning and Development department to deliver the training classes. Other localities could easily replicate with strategy, such as by accessing free or low-cost training in lead-safe work practices.

Contact for Specific Information
Vanessa McCleary
Manager
Community Development Division
Rocky Mount Planning and Development Department
252-972-1100
mccleary@ci.rocky-mount.nc.us

References for additional information
1. Rocky Mount Community Development Division
   www.ci.rocky-mount.nc.us/planning/commdev.html

EQUIP COMMUNITY-BASED ORGANIZATIONS AND SERVICE PROVIDERS

DESCRIPTION OF THE STRATEGY

Training those who provide services to families in high-risk neighborhoods can leverage existing relationships and create a strong infrastructure of leaders and parents who are knowledgeable about lead poisoning. The staff of social service organizations and leaders of community-based organizations (CBOs) are well-positioned to teach their clients and constituents about lead poisoning and means of prevention. The extent of instruction can range from brief orientations to a day-long seminar on topics such as: lead-based paint hazards and prevention; relevant legal rights (including the federal lead hazard disclosure law); and direct service strategies for assisting families of children at risk for lead poisoning.

BENEFITS

Immediate/Direct Results: High-risk families who receive services from the service provider or are the CBOs' constituents will benefit from enhanced knowledge and referrals.

Public Health Benefits: Over time, individual or community-wide actions to protect children from lead exposure may become more commonplace as the staff of the service providers and CBOs teach others about lead hazards and lead poisoning.

Other Indirect/Collateral Benefits: A community that is broadly educated about lead hazards and aware of appropriate preventive measures may be better poised to support programs and policies that advance primary prevention.

SCOPE OF POTENTIAL IMPACT

City- or County-Wide
Neighborhood/Community

PRIMARY ACTORS
Health Department
Community-based Organizations

KEY PARTNERS
Housing Agency
Human Services or Welfare Agency
HUD
Tenants
Volunteers
Community Members

CRITICAL ELEMENTS

Staff requirements: Depends on the number and frequency of training events being offered.

Other resource requirements: The sponsoring agency must have access to means of communication with community-based organizations and service providers to market the training and recruit trainees.

Institutional capacity required: Credibility of the training organization among target audiences is a critical institutional prerequisite.

Cost considerations: Since relevant training materials to serve as models are available in abundance, the major cost consideration is covering staff time and out-of-pocket expenses to deliver the training, such as copying related materials.

Timing issues: Can be implemented at will; however, experienced staff report that a regular ongoing schedule of training sessions offers considerable advantages with respect to recruiting and logistics.

Feasibility of Implementation: High. Strategy is quite feasible in most locales

POTENTIAL OBSTACLES/BARRIERS

It may be difficult to secure funding for such training programs. Organizations and agencies will need to repeat trainings due to staff turnover.

ADDITIONAL RESOURCES

N/A

ILLUSTRATION OF STRATEGY IN PRACTICE

New Jersey Citizen Action offers regular "Train the Trainer" sessions on lead poisoning prevention for staff of social service agencies and community-based organizations (CBOs) who work with high-risk families. Attendees learn about lead poisoning hazards and their prevention; ways to help clients understand their legal, housing, and educational rights; and strategies for assisting families of children at risk for lead poisoning. They also receive assistance in preparing presentations on lead and are encouraged to teach others about lead poisoning prevention. Training dates are set well in advance so that staff can routinely spread the word about upcoming training opportunities. The training is open to anyone, lasts for one day, includes lunch, and is provided at no charge to attendees. Training is usually provided at consistent locations with convenient parking, to make the logistics simple for both attendees and program staff. NJ Citizen Action receives competitive grant funding of about $20,000 per year from the State Department of Human Services, Office of Prevention of Mental Retardation and Developmental Disabilities, to support the training program.

Jurisdiction or Target Area: Newark, New Jersey area

Primary Actor: New Jersey Citizen Action

Secondary Actor(s): N/A

Staffing utilized: NJ Citizen Action tries to include guest speakers, such as attorneys, pediatricians, or parents of lead poisoned children, to avoid the monotony of a single speaker and to provide expert information.

Other resources utilized: Each trainee receives a large binder full of relevant reference materials, including transparencies for use with overhead projectors and a script on lead poisoning designed to make it easier for attendees to become trainers. The training includes lunch.

Factors essential to implementation: NJ Citizen Action staff believe that the most essential factor to continued success of the training is the quality of the training, as attendance would surely fall off if agency managers and CBOs did not perceive value in dedicating a full day of a new staff member's time. Keeping logistics routine enables program staff to focus more on recruiting and providing quality training and outreach than on, for example, catering or parking arrangements.

Limitations/challenges/problems encountered: None listed.

Magnitude of Impact/Potential Impact: Trainees represent a range of entities, including, but not limited to, community-based organizations, day care center staff, tenant groups, school nurses, Head Start staff, union members, city and state agencies, and private health plans. Nearly 200 people were trained in 2003. Feedback from responses to a follow-up form suggests that many trainees share information garnered from the training through newsletters, presentations, and community meetings.

Potential for replication: High.

Contact for Specific Information

New Jersey Citizen Action
732-246-4772

References for additional information

1. NJ Citizen Action is willing to share copies of the training manuals, including the presentation overheads and scripts, to interested programs.

EQUIP DAY LABORERS TO WORK SAFELY

DESCRIPTION OF THE STRATEGY

Research makes clear that routine work disturbing painted surfaces can create lead dust hazards. "Basic training" in lead-safe work practices is now readily available to teach painters, remodelers, and maintenance staff the modest changes in work practices that are needed to control, contain, and clean up any lead dust generated by their work.

Day laborers are typically hired by building contractors for a low hourly wage (with no benefits) and assigned low-skill tasks, such as demolishing and removing dilapidated building components and scraping loose paint. Training in lead-safe work practices (LSWP) will increase the possibility that these workers will protect themselves and their children from lead dust hazards.

It is crucial that delivery of this training be targeted to the increasingly immigrant and non-English-speaking day laborer population who staff the "front line" of repair and rehab work, so that they will know why and how to work safely in all jobs. Immigrant/refugee relief programs, rural assistance programs, and human rights organizations can help locate this population and market lead safety training to them.

BENEFITS

Immediate/Direct Results: Training day laborers to work in a lead-safe manner will result in a reduction in lead dust hazards created due to rehab, repainting, and renovation of pre-1978 housing. Increased awareness in immigrant communities of the relationship between housing and health, and lead hazards specifically, will be a direct result of efforts to train day laborers to work safely.

Public Health Benefits: From a public health perspective, training day laborers to use lead-safe work practices will result in reduced exposure to lead by both families whose homes are being painted or renovated, and the families of day laborers through prevention of the dispersal of lead dust and paint from track-in on the clothes and shoes of the worker.

Other Indirect/Collateral Benefits: Day laborers increase their own power over their health by demanding the right to use lead-safe work practices to protect clients, themselves, and their families.

SCOPE OF POTENTIAL IMPACT

Statewide   Regional (e.g. multi-county)
City- or County-Wide   Neighborhood/Community
Specific (Targeted) Population—Day Laborers

PRIMARY ACTORS	KEY PARTNERS
Health Department	Property Owners
Code or Building Inspection Agency	Contractors
Community-based Organizations	
Day Laborers	

CRITICAL ELEMENTS

Staff requirements: Minimum 0.25 FTE plus time for trainers.

Other resource requirements: Partnerships with Labor Occupational Health and Safety (LOSH) centers.

Institutional capacity required: Experienced bilingual trainer(s) required. Using the "train the trainer" model is most effective in orienting new trainers since peer-to-peer education can continue beyond the scope and funding stream of the program.

Cost considerations: Cost for equipment and sufficient materials for the number of workers to be trained should be considered.

Timing issues: Two to three years may be needed to develop and complete a comprehensive program.

Feasibility of Implementation: Moderate

POTENTIAL OBSTACLES/BARRIERS

The obstacles to delivering a lead-safe work practices training to non-English speaking immigrant communities are many and varied. Skilled, culturally-competent trainers are need to teach the Spanish version of the HUD-EPA course *Lead Safety for Remodeling, Repair and Painting*. The course has not yet been translated into languages needed by non-Spanish speaking immigrants who may also be working as day laborers and at risk for lead hazard exposure. Since many immigrants may not have been able to attend school in their country of origin long enough to equip them to sit through a long, classroom-style training, delivery needs to be paced or staged and include hands-on practices.

The main obstacle to getting day laborers to *use* lead-safe work practices is that the relationship between day laborers and their employers is not conducive to the workers changing work methods based on law and safety. Simply providing a training opportunity for workers is not enough—employers must be motivated or required to comply with lead safety requirements.

ADDITIONAL RESOURCES

1. The HUD/EPA 5½-hour training course includes valuable hands-on exercises and is available in Spanish.
   www.hud.gov/offices/lead/training/rrp/rrp_course.cfm
2. Free training in LSWP is available across the country under the Attorneys General agreement with the National Paint and Coatings Association (NPCA). www.leadsafetraining.org
3. HUD's lead-safe housing rule requires training when performing work that disturbs paint in federally-assisted pre-1978 housing.
   www.hud.gov/offices/lead/leadsaferule/index.cfm
4. Arellano, G, "Diary of a Day Laborer: A human drama in 5 parts", *Orange County Weekly*.
   www.ocweekly.com/ink/01/50/cover-arellano.php

ILLUSTRATION OF STRATEGY IN PRACTICE

In 1999, UCLA's Center for the Study on Urban Poverty estimated that about 20,000 day laborers work in more than 90 sites in Los Angeles and Orange counties. An estimated 98 percent of these workers are from Mexico or Central America; about 95 percent of them enter illegally. Since 1999, that number has continued to grow.

In the face of these trends, the Healthy Homes Outreach Project in Los Angeles has trained over 200 mostly non-English speaking workers, primarily from Mexico and Central America. At four day laborer job centers in Los Angeles and Hollywood, community organizers distributed flyers introducing basic information about lead hazards and the purpose and logistics of the training and recruited training participants. The training was delivered at the day laborer job centers because the sites were well-known to the target audience and because workers who could not find work that day would be readily available to participate. Some workers who previously committed to attending the training could not attend because they found work on the day training was provided and could not afford to miss a rare job opportunity.

This project worked with Labor Occupational Safety and Health (LOSH) centers at University of California–Berkeley and University of California–Los Angeles, which provided worker education around hazards including lead, asbestos, and chemicals. The LOSH partners also educated day laborers on their rights and OSHA requirements and violations.

Funding for this project was provided by a small, local private foundation. Respirators distributed to class participants were purchased with funds from another California-based foundation.

Jurisdiction or Target Area: Los Angeles, CA

Primary Actors: Healthy Homes Collaborative of Southern California, Instituto de Educacion Popular de Sur California (IDEPSCA), Coalition for Humane Immigrant Rights of Los Angeles (CHIRLA)

Secondary Actor(s): LOSH – UC Berkeley, LOSH – UCLA

Staffing utilized: 2 FTE organizers recruited and followed up with workers.

Other resources utilized: Respirators, trainers, training facilities, Spanish language capabilities

Factors essential to implementation: In Los Angeles, healthy homes advocates have found that several steps are needed to successfully deliver the Spanish-language version of the lead-safe work practices course to day laborers. Most day laborers are unable to give up a full 8-hour workday in order to attend training for which they are not compensated. Therefore, advocates have divided the training into several evening sessions. Second, trainers emphasize the self-protective benefits of lead safety, since linking the issue to worker protection has been an important step in engaging day laborers in the issue of lead-safety and in how to prevent hazards in the first place. Third, using written materials as little as possible, and relying on face-to-face explanations and hands-on use of equipment has been the most successful teaching method.

Limitations/challenges/problems encountered: The main barrier to getting day laborers to *use* lead safe work practices is the employer. Given the scarcity of work for a growing population of workers, day laborers are unwilling to raise concern over lead safety with their employers, if they are even aware of this issue. Community and union organizers need to support workers in protecting themselves and their families by "blowing the whistle" on employers circumventing lead safety laws in order to get work done as quickly and cheaply as possible without regard to the health and safety of either the family whose home is being painted or repaired or the family of the worker.

Magnitude of actual impact: The project trained 200 workers in one year. Since a typical day laborer works on an average of 50-100 homes annually, this training has added lead-safe work practices to thousands of projects.

Potential for replication: Moderate. Replica (modified) projects have or are being carried out in several other immigrant communities in the United States, including the Mission District in San Francisco, CA. Every "replication" of this project will vary due to local political, population, and socio-economic variances. This project can most successfully be replicated where lead-safe work practices are required during painting and remodeling activities.

Contacts for Specific Information

Linda Kite
Coordinator
Healthy Homes Collaborative of Southern California
213-689-9170
Lkite@psr.org

Pablo Alvarado
Coordinator
Day Labor Project CHIRLA
213-353-1333
apabloalvarado@aol.com

References for additional information

1. www.chirla.org/programs.htm
2. www.dph.sf.ca.us/ehs/enviro_times/archives/Nov2002/dl_osh_training.htm

EXPAND WEATHERIZATION AND REHAB PROGRAMS TO ADDRESS LEAD SAFETY

DESCRIPTION OF THE STRATEGY

Supplementing weatherization and housing rehab activities in high-risk housing to include targeted lead hazard control activities is an effective, low-cost strategy to address lead hazards in the home and expand the rehab and weatherization crews' knowledge of lead safety. St. Paul (MN) has enhanced standard weatherization efforts with low cost window-focused lead hazard control steps in pre-1978 residential units housing a child under age six. Similar initiatives are underway in California, Indiana, Montana, and Washington.

BENEFITS

Immediate/Direct Results: These efforts offer enormous potential to bring primary prevention to low-income families in older homes whose children are at high risk for lead poisoning. The direct result can be the repair/control of lead hazards before a child is poisoned.

Public Health Benefits: Efforts to proactively fix lead hazards have a significant public health benefit. Repairing windows in older homes undergoing weatherization will reduce lead hazards to children in those homes. Similar efforts to integrate lead into existing rehabilitation programs help reduce exposure to deteriorated lead paint and friction surfaces on windows, both of which are lead hazards.

Other Indirect/Collateral Benefits: These collaborations bring an increased awareness of lead hazards to weatherization and rehab programs. This affects the work that they do even when they are not actively controlling a lead hazard and can result in more attention to lead safe work practices. For example, the MN project which requires dust clearance testing after window treatment work to address lead hazards has helped instill in the contractors the importance of controlling, containing, and cleaning lead dust so that they can pass clearance. Skills and lessons learned about controlling lead dust increase workers' understanding of what it takes to minimize lead dust in jobs where clearance may not be required (e.g., a weatherization or other job with window replacement).

SCOPE OF POTENTIAL IMPACT

Citywide, Regional, or Statewide—If funds are available to support the added lead hazard reduction actions and there is support from state weatherization or rehab program managers.

Specific (Targeted) Population—Low-income families living in older homes. Concentrating on homes with young children increases immediate health benefits.

PRIMARY ACTOR	KEY PARTNERS
Housing Agency	Health Department
Community Action Agency	Community Development Corporations
Health Department	Property Owners
	Weatherization and Housing Rehab Contractors and Workers

CRITICAL ELEMENTS

Staff requirements: The resources required are somewhat related to the scale of the project. In a city or county, an existing weatherization program could partner with a lead hazard control program and, with a percentage of a full time employee's time, structure a project to target weatherization units for lead hazard control. If a broader effort is envisioned to add a lead hazard control element to statewide weatherization or rehab programs, a more substantial commitment of staff resources and funding would be needed.

Other resource requirements: The weatherization program would need equipment and trained personnel to conduct lead inspections and/or risk assessments (to confirm the presence of lead based paint) and perform dust clearance testing. They would also need access to trained and qualified contractors to perform the work.

Institutional capacity required: Typically it is not necessary to change laws or regulations to integrate the delivery of weatherization and lead hazard control services. The main capacity issue is the availability of qualified personnel to perform the hazard assessments (or measure lead content in paint), complete the work following lead safety standards, and conduct clearance tests. Weatherization and rehab programs can have their existing crews perform lead hazard reduction provided they are properly qualified. For abatement projects, workers and contractors must be trained and certified. Except in a few states, training in lead-safe work practices is sufficient qualification for most non-abatement projects. Certified lead inspectors, risk assessors and—in some states—sampling technicians can perform the dust clearance testing after the work is completed.

Cost considerations: Leveraging other programs' work in homes to tackle lead hazards is generally cost effective. Weatherization and rehab programs already bear the costs of identifying housing units appropriate for their programs and their eligibility criteria are consistent with risk indicators for lead hazards (homes built before 1950; low-income families). Expanded programs can therefore offer lead hazard control, building upon existing efforts to enroll units and fix other problems, many of which may also be contributing to lead hazards, such as plumbing leaks, holes in the exterior walls or roof, and poor insulation resulting in condensation and water damage. In some cases, it may be appropriate to purchase XRF machines to help identify homes where lead hazard control is not needed.

Timing issues: If funding is available to support the lead hazard control interventions, approximately 6-12 months is needed to launch such a program. If funding is not reliable, then a more substantial commitment of staff resources and time may be need to structure the appropriate partnerships.

Feasibility of Implementation: Moderate. Implementation can hinge on the availability of dedicated funds to support the added lead work. Weatherization and publicly supported rehab programs generally have production targets that provide disincentives to increasing the costs in individual units. There may also be restrictions on spending the program's funds for actions not directly related to the program's mission (e.g., non-energy based repairs are ineligible for weatherization funding, except that in some states up to 10% can be spent on "health and safety" repairs). A key to implementation therefore is locating funds that can be used for lead work and securing a commitment from the state and local housing and weatherization program managers that this supplemental work is a valuable complement to their central mission.

POTENTIAL OBSTACLES/BARRIERS

Lack of support from the key energy or housing agency staff and/or the local or state lead program can hinder efforts. Funding for added lead work must be secured.

ADDITIONAL RESOURCES
N/A

ILLUSTRATION OF STRATEGY IN PRACTICE

The Department of Public Health supplements weatherization activities in pre-1978 housing with a child under age six to include targeted lead hazard control activities. Window wells are capped and a thorough cleaning of windowsills and floors is completed using a wet wash and HEPA vacuum. Pre- and post-intervention dust samples are collected to document the decline in lead-contaminated dust and to verify that the unit meets dust clearance standards. Clearance testing is performed by certified lead risk assessors. Funding for the lead supplement to the weatherization is provided by a HUD-funded lead hazard reduction grant.

Jurisdiction or Target Area: Ramsey County, Minnesota

Primary Actor: Jim Yannarelly, Ramsey County Department of Public Health, 555 Cedar Street, St. Paul, MN 55101-2260

Secondary Actor(s): N/A

Staffing utilized: The initial staffing required to get the program off the ground was provided in-kind by the HUD funded lead program that is a key partner. Once in place, the program uses existing weatherization staff to conduct the lead hazard control work. They received two days of training which is more extensive than the current one-day Lead Safe Work Practices course required by DOE for weatherization staff. A certified risk assessor completes the clearance testing.

Other resources utilized: The additional per-unit cost of the lead supplement to the weatherization program is approximately $300 for lead hazard control and $150 for clearance testing. It is funded through Minnesota's lead hazard control grant from HUD. Window well caps have been installed in 7 to 15 windows in the unit. Health department staff estimates that the additional cleaning work takes approximately four hours for a two-person crew.

Factors essential to implementation: Funding such as support from the state or regional weatherization program and the HUD lead hazard control grant program or other sources to underwrite the lead treatments is key. Another potential source of funding could be state energy consortiums that are funded by electric utilities to help justify window treatments. The weatherization program must also have policies to ensure the appropriate lead training, work practices, and that clearance testing occurs.

Limitations/challenges/problems encountered: The most difficult aspect of the program is managing the logistics of the various components. A second challenge is the inherent difficulty in proving that such prevention-based action works. The program did not have funds to collect data to document this. Finally, the majority of homes treated by a typical weatherization program are not occupied by a family with a young child.

Magnitude of Impact/Potential Impact: The program targets neighborhoods and homes with key risk factors for lead hazards (older homes built before 1950; low income families which are eligible for weatherization services). To date the program has completed the lead treatments in 61 units, all of which had at least one child under age 6. Slightly more than half of the units were owner-occupied. Health department staff believes that this initiative has helped prevent elevated blood lead levels in units where work occurred. None of the homes were occupied by children with elevated blood lead levels when this work occurred. Contractors performing weatherization now understand how to complete lead dust removal during final cleanup and recognize the importance of controlling lead-contaminated dust. These changes in cleaning behavior extend to jobs in older homes even when there is not a lead specification.

Potential for replication: High. Replicable with willing partners and funding.

Contact for Specific Information
Jim Yannerelly
Lead Program
Ramsey County Department of Public Health
651-266-1280
Jim.Yannarelly@CO.RAMSEY.MN.US

References for additional information
N/A

HOLD REGULAR LEAD-SAFE WORK PRACTICES TRAININGS

DESCRIPTION OF THE STRATEGY

Systematic, ongoing lead safety training opportunities can remove barriers to safe remediation. Agencies that conduct regular training in lead-safe work practices for property owners, including those cited for code violations, will remove the often-utilized excuse that "no training is available." Where other delivery systems are absent, health department personnel may be able to conduct such lead-safe work practices trainings.

BENEFITS

Immediate/Direct Results: Property owners will be provided additional opportunities to be trained in lead-safe work practices.

Public Health Benefits: As more property owners are trained in lead-safe work practices, creation or exacerbation of lead-based paint hazards will decrease, lowering the risk of childhood exposure to lead hazards.

Other Indirect/Collateral Benefits: If required for property owners cited for code violations, this strategy can provide a useful, alternative enforcement mechanism. Instead of levying fines which may never be paid, an enforcement agency can put primary prevention tools in the hands of those who need them most.

SCOPE OF POTENTIAL IMPACT

Statewide   City- or County-Wide
Neighborhood/Community

PRIMARY ACTORS

Health Department
Housing Agency

KEY PARTNERS

Property Owners
Contractors
Painters
Paint Manufacturers
Homeowners

CRITICAL ELEMENTS

Staff requirements: This strategy is not staff-intensive. An experienced trainer will be needed one or two days a month.

Other resource requirements: Lead-safe work practices training materials will be necessary.

Institutional capacity required: Where applicable, instructors certified or accredited in lead-safe work practices training will be required.

Cost considerations: This strategy will incur modest costs by running an ongoing training program. Costs to property owners will be minimal or non-existent.

Timing issues: This strategy will require planning and organization, especially if coordination among state or local agencies is involved. After initial implementation, however, training courses can be offered at any time. Departments or organizations facilitating training projects may find that evening and weekend trainings are better attended.

Feasibility of Implementation: Very high. Training strategies are generally very feasible.

POTENTIAL OBSTACLES/BARRIERS

Tying lead-safe work practices training to code enforcement may prove to be a challenge in some jurisdictions, as enforcement agencies may prefer to rely exclusively on fines. There may also be a lack of interest in ongoing training programs on the part of property owners, or a lack of time to attend such training.

ADDITIONAL RESOURCES

N/A

ILLUSTRATION OF STRATEGY IN PRACTICE

The Alameda County Lead Poisoning Prevention Program conducts a regular schedule of lead-safe painting and remodeling classes, along with a more extensive class in lead-safe work practices.

The introductory lead-safe painting and remodeling classes are free and open to the general public. They are held once a month for two hours and offer simple solutions that property owners can use to repair and renovate their homes. The classes are taught by expert trainers but are not HUD-approved training courses.

The more extensive classes are also held regularly, with two of the monthly classes offered in Spanish. These classes are conducted over the course of an entire day and are recommended for remodelers, renovators, painters, and maintenance workers doing painting and minor repairs. The classes lead to a Notice of Completion in training for lead-safe work practices and meet the minimum training requirements for individuals performing certain activities in federally assisted housing including Section 8. The cost of the classes is $125.

Jurisdiction or Target Area: Alameda County, California

Primary Actor: Alameda County Lead Poisoning Prevention Program

Secondary Actor(s): N/A

Staffing utilized: 0.5 FTE is required for this strategy, including the time of the trainers.

Other resources utilized: N/A

Factors essential to implementation: Having knowledgeable staff on hand and a high level of interest in training classes has been essential to the implementation of this strategy.

Limitations/challenges/problems encountered: There were no significant challenges or problems.

Magnitude of Impact/Potential Impact: 238 individuals have been trained in the more extensive lead-safe work practices through March 2004. Also in 2004, ACLPPP provided the one-day lead-safety training to 100-120 day laborers. ACLPPP does not maintain detailed data on the number of people trained through the informal, two-hour introductory course.

Potential for replication: The potential for replication is high.

Contact for Specific Information

Dennis Jordan
Director, Alameda County Lead Poisoning Prevention Program
510-567-8280

References for additional information

N/A

PROVIDE TECHNICAL ASSISTANCE TO PROPERTY OWNERS

DESCRIPTION OF THE STRATEGY

Cities, states, and community-based organizations can provide technical assistance to property owners who are seeking to meet lead-safe housing and lead hazard control requirements or to voluntarily implement lead safety measures. As a complement to relevant training in lead-safe work practices and regulatory requirements, individualized technical assistance can accelerate the pace at which property owners and contractors retool the way they work. Depending on the scope of the strategy, technical assistance can be accessible through a hotline, one-on-one visits at a "one-stop" center, or a user-friendly interactive website.

BENEFITS

Immediate/Direct Results: Providing individualized assistance in meeting lead-safe housing requirements can accelerate the pace at which property owners and their contractors adopt lead-safe work practices and complete lead hazard control work.

Public Health Benefits: Expediting the adoption of lead-safe work practices and the completion of lead hazard control work will protect children who might otherwise be exposed to lead hazards.

Other Indirect/Collateral Benefits: Local and state government agencies will develop new relationships and chains of communication with property owners and contractors in the course of delivering technical assistance. In the process, these agencies, which may normally be seen as antagonistic toward property owners, will learn about the issues and needs facing the owners of high-risk housing and be able to address gaps in their understanding of lead safety. Also, the property owners will be better positioned to successfully assume their role as partners in the effort to prevent childhood lead poisoning.

SCOPE OF POTENTIAL IMPACT

Statewide   Regional
City- or County-Wide

PRIMARY ACTORS

Health Department
Housing Agency
Community-based Organizations

KEY PARTNERS

Property Owners
Homeowners

CRITICAL ELEMENTS

Staff requirements: Staff requirements will vary substantially based upon the scope of the strategy. Some small projects may only require 1-2 FTE, while larger projects may need a staff of 6 or more FTE to properly engage property owners on an individualized basis.

Other resource requirements: N/A

Institutional capacity required: This strategy requires staff knowledgeable in lead safety and state and federal lead standards. Staff members with the ability to relate to and work cooperatively with property owners are also essential.

Cost considerations: Costs to administer this strategy will depend on scope, but could be significant due to the individualized nature of the strategy. The largest costs to the agency or organization implementing the strategy will come from staff salaries.

Timing issues: There are no distinct timing issues with this strategy.

Feasibility of Implementation: High. This strategy can be implemented and administered with a moderate amount of effort.

POTENTIAL OBSTACLES/BARRIERS

The main potential obstacle or barrier to implementing this strategy will be a lack of funding for project staff. States and localities with tight budgets will need to look for creative funding mechanisms to implement their specific technical assistance projects.

ADDITIONAL RESOURCES

N/A

ILLUSTRATION OF STRATEGY IN PRACTICE

Rhode Island's Lead Hazard Mitigation law requires the state to provide technical assistance to property owners who seek to comply with the law requiring the repair of lead hazards using lead safe work practices and clearance. The Housing Resources Commission is charged with crafting and implementing a technical assistance plan. When the plan is fully implemented, the state will provide property owners with access to technical service centers. These centers will be "one-stop shops" where owners will be able to gain hands-on experience with lead hazard mitigation, work one-on-one with technical assistance staff, and find resources on how to obtain financial assistance for making their properties lead-safe. It is anticipated that the state will have these centers in place by July 1, 2005.

Jurisdiction or Target Area: Rhode Island

Primary Actor: Housing Resources Commission

Secondary Actor(s): N/A

Staffing utilized: To fully implement the program, the Housing Resources Commission estimates it will need 6 FTE.

Other resources utilized: N/A

Factors essential to implementation: Factors essential to implementation include the ability to secure funding for technical assistance staff, as well as property owners' use of the technical assistance resources.

Limitations/challenges/problems encountered: Without funding, the Housing Resources Commission will not be able to retain sufficient technical assistance staff.

Magnitude of Impact/Potential Impact: The technical assistance plan has not yet been implemented. However, the state expects many property owners to use its technical assistance resources as they work to meet the requirements of Rhode Island's lead hazard mitigation law.

Potential for replication: Given the availability of professionals able to provide technical assistance regarding lead-safe work practices and lead hazard control, this strategy is fairly easy to replicate.

Contact for Specific Information
Simon Kue
Rhode Island Housing Resources Commission
401-450-1349
www.HRC.ri.gov

TRAIN AND EMPLOY LOW-INCOME COMMUNITY RESIDENTS IN HAZARD CONTROL

DESCRIPTION OF THE STRATEGY

Environmental health services can be provided to communities through programs that train and employ low-income community residents, including parents of lead-poisoned children and parents of children at high risk. The services provided can consist of low-cost hazard control, cleaning, peer education, and the provision of products that reduce environmental health hazards. Health departments, housing agencies, and community-based organizations can work independently or collaboratively to provide these trainings.

BENEFITS

Immediate/Direct Results: Where demand for services exist, low-income residents will have the opportunity to obtain steady, meaningful employment and will be trained to recognize and control lead hazards in their own homes. These residents will likely relate well to other low-income families in their area, supporting hazard control and peer education efforts. Hazard control and other services will also be available to low-income property owners and tenants who may not have had access to such services in the past.

Public Health Benefits: Providing low-cost services like hazard control can increase the number of hazards reduced in a particular community, leading to greater primary prevention of childhood lead poisoning.

Other Indirect/Collateral Benefits: This strategy can help reduce unemployment in a local area and can be one useful tool used to combat poverty. Low-income residents will also gain work skills that they may not have been able to obtain elsewhere.

SCOPE OF POTENTIAL IMPACT

City- or County-Wide   Neighborhood/Community

PRIMARY ACTORS	KEY PARTNERS
Health Department	Property Owners
Housing Agency	Tenants
Community-based Organizations	Parents
	Community Members

CRITICAL ELEMENTS

Staff requirements: This will vary on the scope of the strategy. If the project will involve employing low-income workers, new staff will be required.

Other resource requirements: Trainers, educational materials, and environmental health products may be required, depending on the scope of the strategy.

Institutional capacity required: Some projects undertaken by local government agencies may need prior city council/county board approval.

Cost considerations: Overall costs will depend on the scope of the strategy. Projects that involve employing community residents will have higher costs than those that provide training or environmental health products.

Timing issues: This strategy will require some planning and good organization; projects involving employing community residents will also require some lead time for the hiring process.

Feasibility of Implementation: High. This strategy should be feasible to implement.

POTENTIAL OBSTACLES/BARRIERS

In some areas, projects that involve employing community residents may find a lack of potential employees. Other challenges to this type of project could include employee retention problems.

ADDITIONAL RESOURCES

N/A

ILLUSTRATION OF STRATEGY IN PRACTICE

Healthy Homes Services is a program of The Way Home (TWH), a non-profit tenant rights and social services agency in Manchester, New Hampshire. The program trains and employs low-income community residents, including parents of lead-poisoned children and children at high risk, to provide environmental health services to their communities. These services, which include low-cost hazard control, peer education, and the provision of products that reduce environmental health hazards, have proven to be one way to advance primary prevention efforts.

Jurisdiction or Target Area: Manchester, New Hampshire

Primary Actor: The Way Home/Healthy Homes Services

Secondary Actor(s): N/A

Staffing utilized: Healthy Homes Services has 3 FTE staff.

Other resources utilized: The Healthy Homes Services project was initially launched under a small grant from the U.S. Environmental Protection Agency. Currently, the project is operating as a sub-grantee to the City of Manchester, under a substantial HUD Lead Hazard Control grant. Staff knowledgeable in lead safety, peer education, and training low-income residents have also been utilized by the project.

Factors essential to implementation: A dedicated source of funding and interest from landlords and residents have been essential to implementing this strategy.

Limitations/challenges/problems encountered: Reliance on grants and low-interest loans are challenges the project has faced. The project is now seeking to become sustainable through small contracts and offering more services at low cost, which will allow it to operate without heavy reliance on grants.

Magnitude of Impact/Potential Impact: As of the beginning of 2004, the project had trained a total of 31 low-income residents, seven in peer education and 24 in low-cost lead hazard control.

Potential for replication: Moderate. Initially, any project similar to Healthy Homes Services will rely on grant funding. With a commitment to use initial grant money to seek out other sustainable funding, this strategy has a high potential for replication.

Contact for Specific Information
Mary Sliney
Executive Director, The Way Home
603-627-5403

References for additional information
N/A

COLLABORATIONS, PARTNERSHIPS, AND INCENTIVES

COLLABORATE FOR LEAD SAFETY IN CHILD CARE HOMES

CREATE INCENTIVES TO INTEGRATE LEAD SAFETY INTO HOUSING REHABILITATION

INTRODUCE INCENTIVES FOR LEAD SAFETY INTO CHILD CARE PROGRAMS

LEND OUT LEAD SAFETY EQUIPMENT

SHARE RISK ASSESSMENT AND LEAD SAMPLING SERVICES

TEACH CODE INSPECTORS ABOUT LEAD SAFETY THROUGH JOINT VISITS

COLLABORATE FOR LEAD SAFETY IN CHILD CARE HOMES

DESCRIPTION OF THE STRATEGY

Protecting children in child care settings is an essential complement to preventing exposure in the home environment. Using collaborations between local child care providers, associations that represent their interests, and local housing or health agencies can ensure that child care homes (i.e. child care based in the private home of the caregiver) are renovated to provide a lead-safe and healthy environment in which children thrive.

BENEFITS

Immediate/Direct Results: Participating child care homes will have facilities that are lead-safe and healthier for children.

Public Health Benefits: If a child care home has lead hazards, many children may become lead poisoned. Since the children served may not otherwise be considered at high risk for lead poisoning, they may not be identified under targeted screening programs. Reducing lead hazards in these facilities will benefit all of the children who use the child care homes' services. Awareness of healthy homes approaches in the properties where their children spend time may prompt parents to consider like measures in their own homes. If child care homes are similar to all homes, they are almost twice as likely to have lead hazards than a licensed, non-home-based child care center.

Other Indirect/Collateral Benefits: The owners of child care homes may be reluctant to address lead hazards given competing priorities. If competitors are marketing their lead-safe and healthy status, they may be more likely to address the issue. They may also be more willing to accept a lead-safe mandate if industry leaders have a model for success to allay fears.

SCOPE OF POTENTIAL IMPACT

There are 14,200 licensed non-home-based, child care centers nationally. There may be as many as ten times more child care homes that are not licensed.

City- or County-Wide
Neighborhood/Community
Specific (Targeted) Population—The approach may be expanded to non-home based child care centers but HUD funding may be more limited.

PRIMARY ACTORS	KEY PARTNERS
Housing Agency	Health Department
Child Care Providers	Community-based Organizations
	Property Owners
	Parents

CRITICAL ELEMENTS

Staff requirements: One FTE will be needed to establish and manage the program and conduct outreach to the proprietors of child care homes. The amount of time depends on the number of providers to be solicited to participate in the program. A small community might not need a full-time person while a large area with many unlicensed child care homes may need more staff.

Other resource requirements: A strong association representing the child care providers, especially the home-based providers, is extremely helpful. The association can market the opportunity and provide the basic education needed to have willing and able participants.

Institutional capacity required: Qualified personnel are needed to check for hazards and make repairs. In many states, a lead sampling technician can check for deteriorated paint and lead dust hazards. If the home is pre-1950 or lead hazards are suspected, a risk assessment should be performed to check for hazards and determine what is needed to make the property lead-safe. It would be beneficial if the sampling technician or risk assessor were familiar with asthma triggers and methods to reduce those sources since asthma is a significant concern for most child care providers. Contractors or workers trained to perform lead hazard control will be needed to perform the work. After work is completed the property must pass a clearance test (performed by a sampling technician in the 23 states where they are clearly authorized, or by a risk assessor).

Cost considerations: Grant or loan money will probably be needed to fund the lead hazard control. The agency that administers the locality's funds from HUD's Community Development Block Grant program is a possible source of funding. Funds awarded by HUD's HOME, Healthy Homes, LEAP, and Lead Hazard Control Programs can also be used for child care homes if the household is income-eligible.

Timing issues: The program can begin quickly once funds are secured. While a collaborative team of stakeholders could be formed after funds are available, the team may have to be established in order to demonstrate capacity to implement the program and secure funding. Child care providers are busiest—and therefore unavailable—during August and September when children return to school and establish enrollment. Work may be scheduled during provider vacations to reduce relocation costs.

Feasibility of Implementation: Moderate. The program is feasible if grant or loan funding is available. Expanding beyond lead hazards to address asthma triggers such as mold, cockroaches, and dust mites may increase acceptance by meeting the growing concern to families and caregivers. Therefore, the program needs to be able to deal with the most relevant mix of addressable environmental hazards. Relocation of the provider's family and the child care business to a temporary location may need to be addressed.

POTENTIAL OBSTACLES/BARRIERS

If communities do not have a broader program to educate potential clients to consider lead safety and healthy homes issues in the selection of a child care home, the broader impact from competition will be lost.

ADDITIONAL RESOURCES

1. National Resource Center for Health and Safety in Child Care—1-800-598-5437
    http://nrc.uchsc.edu
2. Department of Housing and Urban Development
    www.hud.gov/offices/lead/techstudies/NatlChildCareSurvey_V1_Lead.pdf

ILLUSTRATION #1 OF STRATEGY IN PRACTICE

Since 1998, GMDCA launched the Healthy Environment for Early Learning (HEEL) program. The program has completed lead hazard reduction projects on 125 Minneapolis child care homes. GMDCA completed indoor air quality assessments and mitigation on 70 homes. Through HEEL, GMDCA offers a two-hour class called "Where They Live and Breathe" to all child care providers in Hennepin County. Minneapolis is located in Hennepin County. All providers receiving lead hazard control and indoor air quality assessments must complete the class.

Jurisdiction or Target Area: Minneapolis and Hennepin County, Minnesota

Primary Actor: Greater Minneapolis Day Care Association (GMDCA)

Secondary Actor(s): City of Minneapolis for two rounds of Lead Hazard Control Grants and CDBG funding for the Renovation Loan Program. Hennepin County for the latest round of grants.

Staffing utilized: The program is managed by 1 FTE.

Other resources utilized: Two rounds of lead hazard control grants from HUD to the City of Minneapolis funded the work to make homes lead-safe at an average cost (based on the latest round of grants) of $8500 per home. A recent grant from HUD to Hennepin County continues the program and allows limited expansion to suburban providers. The Minneapolis Renovation Loan Program provided Community Development Block Grant program funds for the indoor air quality assessments and mitigation. The indoor air quality assessments and mitigation averaged $2,000 per home.

Factors essential to implementation: Critical factors were Lead Hazard Control and CDBG funding through HUD and a local association willing and able to coordinate the program.

Limitations/challenges/problems encountered: Funding must be available for the work.

Magnitude of Impact/Potential Impact: 125 home-based, child care homes were made lead-safe. 70 home-based, child care homes had reduced asthma triggers.

Potential for replication: Very high.

Contact for Specific Information
Ed Petsche
HEEL Coordinator
612-349-0563
leadpro@gmdca.org

References for additional information
1. Greater Minneapolis Day-Care Association
   www.gmdca.org

ILLUSTRATION #2 OF STRATEGY IN PRACTICE

The program is designed to improve the quality of 25 home-based child care providers serving more than 150 children in Rochester and Syracuse by making them lead-safe and addressing other healthy homes and general safety issues. To avoid disruption to services and protect the children who attend the homes, the program is providing temporary relocation to an alternative location while renovations are underway. The program educates providers and parents using their services on lead poisoning and daily maintenance techniques to reduce lead hazards and other environmental hazards. It is designed to serve as a model for other communities.

Jurisdiction or Target Area: Rochester and Syracuse, New York

Primary Actor: National Center for Healthy Housing (NCHH)

Secondary Actor(s): Rochester Children's Nursery/Family Child Care Satellite Network of Greater Rochester (FCCSN), Child Care Council of Onondaga County (CCCOC), Home HeadQuarters, Inc (HHQ), and Neighborhood Housing Services of Rochester, Inc. (NHSR).

Staffing utilized: NCHH has committed one full-time equivalent person to the project.

Other resources utilized: HUD provided $930,789 for the project. NCHH and its partners raised an additional $325,846.

Factors essential to implementation: HUD Operation Lead Elimination Action Project funding and local associations willing and able to coordinate the program.

Limitations/challenges/problems encountered: None.

Magnitude of Impact/Potential Impact: Up to 150 children will benefit from the creation of 25 safe, healthy, and lead-safe child care homes.

Potential for replication: Very high. The project is producing an implementation guide and document templates so it can be replicated in other communities. Funding must be available for the lead hazard control work.

Contacts for Specific Information

Carol Kawecki
Program Director
410-772-2779
ckawecki@centerforhealthyhousing.org

Patricia Magnuson
212-262-9575 ext 114
pmagnuson@enterprisefoundation.org

References for additional information

1. National Center for Healthy Housing
   www.centerforhealthyhousing.org/html/projects_demonstration.html
2. The Enterprise Foundation
   www.enterprisefoundation.org

CREATE INCENTIVES TO INTEGRATE LEAD SAFETY INTO HOUSING REHABILITATION

DESCRIPTION OF THE STRATEGY

HUD's regulations require that federally assisted housing rehab projects be done lead safely. Lead poisoning prevention programs can support HUD-funded housing agencies' and community development corporations' (CDCs) efforts to ensure compliance by providing training to build capacity and technical assistance to model the practical application of lead-safe housing requirements. They can also provide services such as risk assessments, recommendations for the scope of work that should be performed, and clearance testing after rehab projects are complete. Jurisdictions that have lead hazard control funds can use them as leverage to encourage housing agencies' and CDCs' rehab of homes with lead hazards.

BENEFITS

Immediate/Direct Results: The scope of the community's rehab program is preserved or expanded to incorporate housing units and work items within homes that might not otherwise have been completed. In addition, the work is done using lead-safe work practices, thus protecting the health of children and other occupants.

Public Health Benefits: Fewer lead poisoned children and increased supply of lead-safe housing.

Other Indirect/Collateral Benefits: The training of private contractors in lead-safe work practices will have significant benefits. For instance, contractors can apply lead-safe work practices to all future rehabilitation and repair projects.

SCOPE OF POTENTIAL IMPACT

City- or County-Wide—Can apply to jurisdiction of county or city health department
Neighborhood/Community—Can target specific neighborhoods

PRIMARY ACTORS	KEY PARTNERS
Health Department	Housing Agency
	Community-based Organizations
	Contractors

CRITICAL ELEMENTS

Staff requirements: The staffing needs are minimal.

Other resource requirements: If lead inspections are provided, XRF analyzers will be needed.

Institutional capacity required: State regulatory agencies must take a flexible, practical approach to incorporating lead hazard control into rehab projects. Requiring abatement certification exceeds HUD requirements and may unnecessarily increase the cost of smaller rehab projects. Communities need a combination of certified workers and workers trained in lead-safe work practices to perform large- and small-scale rehab projects respectively.

Cost considerations: First, rehab costs will increase incrementally as a result of contractors using safe work practices and for minor activities such as additional set-up and clean-up steps. Ideally, another funding source should be made available to help pay the additional costs of lead hazard control that are above and beyond the scope of the rehabilitation work. Alternatively, health departments might charge fees to the housing agency for performing lead inspections or risk assessments, as well as training contractors and workers, to support the continuation of skilled staff.

Timing issues: The health department and the housing agency need to agree on the timing of the risk assessment, the housing inspection, and the development of specifications. There are many different approaches, which basically fall into two camps. The first is to develop the rehab scope of work which is then given to the risk assessor. The risk assessment will then suggest additional work required by the risk assessment and specific work practices that should be followed during the rehab. The second is to conduct the risk assessment first so that all lead hazard control work can be incorporated into the rehab scope of work from the outset. Either approach can be effective, but there must be agreement on protocols before launching a collaborative venture.

Feasibility of Implementation: High. This primary prevention strategy can be implemented in communities where there is an interest and a will to make it work. Effective strategic planning for preventing childhood lead poisoning can foster such resource sharing between housing rehab programs and CLPPPS.

POTENTIAL OBSTACLES/BARRIERS

Individual state regulations and requirements can be a barrier. State policy must be flexible while maintaining consistency on basic principles. In addition, a state or local requirement for lead hazard insurance can present an obstacle to getting contractors to perform rehab work.

ADDITIONAL RESOURCES

1. www.hud.gov/offices/lead/leadsaferule/index.cfm

ILLUSTRATION OF STRATEGY IN PRACTICE

The Health Department performs a range of services for community development corporations conducting housing rehab using federal funds. It performs risk assessments, specifies the scope of work for lead hazard control which is incorporated into the rehab specifications, conducts post-work clearance examinations, trains workers in lead-safe work practices (LSWP), and provides up to $2,000 per unit in matching funds for rehab projects. This broad spectrum of services constitutes a powerful incentive for the public and private rehabilitation industry to address lead hazards using lead-safe work practices.

Jurisdiction or Target Area: St. Paul - Ramsey County, Minnesota

Primary Actor: St. Paul – Ramsey County Health Department

Secondary Actor(s): N/A

Staffing Utilized: 0.5 FTE

Other resources utilized: N/A

Factors essential to implementation: A supply of skilled remodeling contractors; close working relationship between the Health Department and multiple community development corporations and agencies managing rehab programs; and an agreed upon protocol for integrating the work of the Health Department and the housing agencies.

Limitations/challenges/problems encountered: The high rate of turnover in the rehab workforce requires repeated delivery of lead-safe work practices training, which helps to integrate LSWP in building trades.

Magnitude of Impact/Potential Impact: Lead hazards are controlled and prevented in approximately 100 units undergoing rehabilitation each year, primarily single family properties and duplexes.

Potential for replication: High, if there is a good working relationship between the various partners.

Contact for Specific Information

Jim Yannarelly
Environmental Health Program Supervisor
651-266-1282
jim.yannarelly@co.ramsey.mn.us

References for additional information

N/A

INTRODUCE INCENTIVES FOR LEAD SAFETY INTO CHILD CARE PROGRAMS

DESCRIPTION OF THE STRATEGY

Protecting children in child care facilities is an essential complement to preventing exposure in the home environment. Providing facilities with marketing and technical assistance through a recognition program can motivate them to reduce lead hazards in the facilities and reduce children's risk of exposure outside the home.

BENEFITS

Immediate/Direct Results: Participating child care programs will go beyond the requirements of the law to address lead hazards.

Public Health Benefits: Reducing lead hazards in these facilities will benefit all of the children who use the child care center's services.

Other Indirect/Collateral Benefits: Child care providers are typically reluctant to address lead hazards in their facilities given competing priorities and resource limitations. They may oppose mandatory requirements. Recognizing leadership on lead safety within the child care community may help allay fears, serve as a model of success, and possibly help facilitate future acceptance of a mandate.

SCOPE OF POTENTIAL IMPACT

There are 100,000 licensed, non-home-based child care facilities nationally. According to the First National Environmental Health Survey of Child Care Centers [Office of Healthy Homes and Lead Hazard Control at the U.S. Department of Housing and Urban Development. First National Environmental Health Survey. Washington, DC; July 15, 2003. Available from URL: www.hud.gov/offices/lead/techstudies/ NatlChildCareSurvey_V1_Lead.pdf. 14 percent of licensed child care facilities in the United States are estimated to have significant lead-based paint hazards—primarily deteriorated lead-based paint. 470,000 children attend these facilities. For facilities in buildings built before 1960, the rate is 26 percent. For facilities where the majority of the children are African American, the rate is 30 percent.

Statewide   City- or County-Wide
Area Covered by Child Care Provider Association(s)

PRIMARY ACTORS	KEY PARTNERS
Health Department	Code or Building Inspection Agency
Human Services Agency	Day Care Providers

CRITICAL ELEMENTS

Staff requirements: Approximately 0.25 FTE for two years to develop and implement the program. Leading child care providers need to participate in the development of the program so that they can support it in the community.

Other resource requirements: A free risk assessment is a strong incentive for child care facilities to consider participating. The sponsoring entity may contract out the risk assessment or use qualified in-house staff. The contractual cost for a risk assessment is about $500 per facility, including $100 for lab costs.

Institutional capacity required: It is helpful to have in-house staff licensed as a lead risk assessor so that a risk assessment can be provided in conjunction with other technical assistance.

Cost considerations: Staff will need to conduct a four-hour site visit to evaluate each facility for lead-based paint hazards and other hazards.

Timing issues: It will take 6-12 months to establish the program, build support for it, and develop materials. Full implementation usually will take an additional year. Child care facilities are busiest—and therefore unavailable—during August and September when children are returning to school or enrolling.

Feasibility of Implementation: Moderate. The program is feasible but to reach the child care facilities most in need of support and oversight, the program should ideally to be part of a larger effort to improve health conditions within all child care facilities. In addition, the program is difficult to implement if narrowly focused on lead hazards. Most child care facilities view asthma triggers such as mold, cockroaches and dust mites as a bigger concern. Therefore, services that address a broad mix of environmental hazards will be more readily accepted.

POTENTIAL OBSTACLES/BARRIERS

Lead hazards are most effectively addressed in the context of a broader evaluation of environmental hazards, especially mold and moisture; pests and pesticides; and carbon monoxide.

Communities need to be prepared to identify potential resources to address lead hazards and provide technical assistance to help facilities obtain and use those resources.

ADDITIONAL RESOURCES

1. National Resource Center for Health and Safety in Child Care at 800-598-5437
    http://nrc.uchsc.edu
2. First National Environmental Health Survey of Child Care Centers by the U.S. Department of Housing and Urban Development
    www.hud.gov/offices/lead/techstudies/NatlChildCareSurvey_V1_Lead.pdf

ILLUSTRATION #1 OF STRATEGY IN PRACTICE

In 1999, IDEM developed a 5-Star Environmental Recognition Program for Child Care Facilities to publicly recognize facilities that go beyond the minimum legal requirements. If the operators or management of the facilities agree to identify and address a variety of environmental hazards, IDEM conducts a no-cost lead risk assessment and provides a comprehensive manual that addresses all compliance requirements related to environmental hazards. In 2002, FSSA modified its regulations for child care centers (larger operations) at 470 IAC 3-4.7-100 to require that peeling paint on any interior or exterior surface or on any equipment be made inaccessible to children if it contains lead until the peeling material is analyzed by a lab and an approved abatement plan is carried out.

Jurisdiction or Target Area: Indiana

Primary Actor: Indiana Department of Environmental Management (IDEM) & Family and Social Service Administration (FSSA) – Child Care Health Section

Secondary Actor(s): N/A

Staffing utilized: 0.25 full-time equivalent staff at IDEM to establish and facilitate program start-up.

Other resources utilized: FSSA added responsibilities to existing inspectors.

Factors essential to implementation: Positive recognition of leadership as well as commitment to providing sustained technical support.

Limitations/challenges/problems encountered: A recognition program typically attracts facilities in good shape; the best practices may only get to implementation at scale after the recognition program has set the stage for a regulatory mandate for the best practices.

Magnitude of Impact/Potential Impact: 41 child care centers, 14 child care homes, and 3 ministry-based child care facilities currently participate in the recognition program.

Potential for replication: High. Readily applicable by any jurisdiction that licenses child care centers.

Contacts for Specific Information

Gayla McCarty
5-Star Program Coordinator
317-233-1046
gmccarty@dem.state.in.us

Gary Rogers
Child Care Inspector
317-233-5412
Grogers@fssa.state.in.us

References for additional information

1. Indiana Department of Environmental Management – 5-Star Environmental Recognition Program for Child-Care Facilities
   www.in.gov/idem/kids/5star/index.html.

ILLUSTRATION #2 OF STRATEGY IN PRACTICE

In 1992, Maine passed a law that requires all licensed child care facilities to have a lead inspection prior to licensing. In 1998, the Maine CLPPP program partnered with the Maine Department of Environmental Protection (DEP) and the Maine Daycare Licensing Bureau to design a workable lead inspection process. All state daycare inspectors conduct a preliminary lead assessment as a prerequisite for licensing. The daycare inspectors use a rated checklist that the Maine CLPPP and DEP programs developed. If the total number on the checklist passes a designated threshold, the daycare inspector orders a full lead inspection by a state-licensed lead inspector.

If a full lead inspection is required, it is scheduled and paid for by the Daycare Licensing Bureau. If lead hazards are identified, the daycare owner is required to abate to at least a lead-safe level. The Daycare Licensing Bureau has some funds available if daycare owners are unable to afford to do the abatement work. To ensure lead safety compliance, state daycare inspectors repeat the preliminary lead assessment as part of an annual daycare inspection for all licensed daycare facilities in Maine.

Jurisdiction or Target Area: Maine

Primary Actor: Maine Childhood Lead Poisoning Prevention Program (CLPPP)

Secondary Actor(s): Maine Department of Environmental Protection; Maine Daycare Licensing Bureau

Staffing utilized: 0.5 FTE.

Other resources utilized: Maine's law was changed in 1998 to allow CLPPP, DEP, and the Daycare Licensing Bureau to carry out this strategy. The Maine approach to this strategy also utilizes a small funding source within the Daycare Licensing Bureau.

Factors essential to implementation: Cooperation from DEP and the Maine Daycare Licensing Bureau and availability of a small funding source were essential to the implementation of this strategy.

Limitations/challenges/problems encountered: The initial resistance to the provision required designing the implementation to accommodate daycare providers' concerns about cost.

Magnitude of Impact/Potential Impact: All licensed daycare centers in Maine are currently in compliance with lead safety standards. The Maine Daycare Licensing Bureau establishes compliance through periodic inspections, with assistance from DEP.

Potential for replication: Moderate. Applicable by any jurisdiction that licenses child care centers and has funding and cooperative partners to help establish and maintain the program.

Contact for Specific Information
MaryAnn Amrich, RN
Program Manager
Childhood Lead Poisoning Prevention Program
Maine Bureau of Health
207-287-8753
MaryAnn.Amrich@maine.gov

References for additional information
N/A

LEND OUT LEAD SAFETY EQUIPMENT

DESCRIPTION OF THE STRATEGY

Communities can promote lead-safe work practices and prevent the creation of lead hazards by making available lead safety equipment for remodeling and renovation at no cost to the borrower. Several jurisdictions around the country have successfully implemented this strategy, most utilizing HEPA vacuums. Including lead-safeequipment used in renovation projects, such as shrouded planers, sanders, and scrapers, in a free loan strategy can make it all the more effective in preventing the creation of lead hazards.

BENEFITS

Immediate/Direct Results: Getting lead safety equipment into the hands of contractors and do-it-yourself renovators makes it possible to reduce the number and severity of lead dust hazards created during remodeling or renovation.

Public Health Benefits: Preventing exposure to lead dust hazards created by remodeling or renovation will reduce the incidence of childhood lead poisoning.

Other Indirect/Collateral Benefits: An equipment loaner program can create opportunities for dialogue and cooperation between public agencies and contractors, landlords, homeowners, and others whose actions disturb painted surfaces.

SCOPE OF POTENTIAL IMPACT

City- or County-Wide   Neighborhood/Community

PRIMARY ACTORS	KEY PARTNERS
Health Department	Community-based Organizations
Housing Agency	Property Owners
	Contractors
	Equipment Suppliers
	Homeowners

CRITICAL ELEMENTS

Staff requirements: No new staff should be required to implement this strategy: a fraction of an existing FTE may be required to support the loan, return, and maintenance of the equipment.

Other resource requirements: Resources needed include the lead safety equipment and staff knowledgeable in the use and maintenance of that equipment. Outside expertise may be required for related staff training. Outreach resources are also needed to promote the availability of the equipment.

Institutional capacity required: Commensurate with the capacity of most health departments and lead hazard control grant programs.

Cost considerations: Costs to administer this strategy will be moderate; actual costs will depend on the scope of the program, i.e. the amount of equipment to be made available.

Timing issues: Implementation should be fairly straightforward once funds and the source of lead safety equipment are approved.

Feasibility of Implementation: Very high. This strategy should be easy to implement and administer.

POTENTIAL OBSTACLES/BARRIERS

There are two potential obstacles to realizing this strategy. First, funding may not be available to purchase the equipment, even though costs to do so will not be prohibitive in most instances. Second, a jurisdiction or an organization may be stymied by the potential for liability exposure.

ADDITIONAL RESOURCES

N/A

ILLUSTRATION OF STRATEGY IN PRACTICE

In 1997, the Manchester Health Department, as part of its overall lead poisoning prevention program, purchased three HEPA vacuums, along with shrouded planers, shrouded scrapers, and shrouded sanders. This equipment is made available through what is known as the Lead Safety Equipment Lending Library for free for use in renovation and remodeling projects that may disturb lead-based paint and that have the potential to create lead hazards. The City also provides some training in the use of the equipment.

Jurisdiction or Target Area: Manchester, CT

Primary Actor: Manchester Health Department

Secondary Actor(s): N/A

Staffing utilized: No new staff was needed to implement this strategy.

Other resources utilized: The Health Department purchased three HEPA vacuums, as well as a shrouded planer, a shrouded scraper, and a shrouded sander. The total cost for all equipment was approximately $3,000.

Factors essential to implementation: The main factor essential to implementation of this strategy was overcoming concerns by the City of Manchester about potential liability issues. The City determined that its insurance would cover any potential liability, allaying concerns.

Limitations/challenges/problems encountered: Again, the greatest challenge here was persuading Manchester than the benefits of the Lending Library far outweighed potential liability.

Magnitude of Impact/Potential Impact: To publicize the Lending Library, the health department placed articles in local news and notified all local hardware stores and paint stores. Since the strategy's inception six years ago, contractors and do-it-yourself renovators have borrowed the equipment for approximately 100 jobs. As Manchester has 9,200 homes or homes built before 1950, the relative usefulness and impact of this strategy has been high.

Potential for replication: Staff at the Manchester Health Department assert that the potential for replication of this strategy is high. Outside of the liability issues already mentioned, this strategy is easy to implement, requiring only an initial equipment purchase and a subsequent tracking system for the equipment as it is loaned out and returned.

Contact for Specific Information

Sue Heller
Manchester Health Department
860-647-3288
Sue41@ci.manchester.ct.us
www.ci.manchester.ct.us/lead/innovations.htm

SHARE RISK ASSESSMENT AND LEAD SAMPLING SERVICES

DESCRIPTION OF THE STRATEGY

Property owners knowledgeable about lead safety can assess other property owners' properties that may have otherwise been ignored. To encourage such exchanges, state and local agencies can provide free training in risk assessment and lead sampling to property owners, with the requirement that those trained perform free risk assessments in other properties, in a type of "good neighbor" program. The property owners would acquire appropriate certificates or licenses after completion of the course.

BENEFITS

Immediate/Direct Results: More property owners will be trained in risk assessment and sampling. The good neighbor component of the strategy also holds potential to substantially increase the number of properties checked for lead-based paint hazards.

Public Health Benefits: Increased risk assessment, lead sampling, and clearance testing will reduce the number of lead hazards to which children are exposed.

Other Indirect/Collateral Benefits: Cooperative working relationships among property owners, and between property owners and regulatory agencies, will be fostered. This should create an environment where hazard reduction and remediation is undertaken on a more voluntary basis with less adversarial enforcement necessary.

SCOPE OF POTENTIAL IMPACT

City- or County-Wide   Neighborhood/Community

PRIMARY ACTORS   KEY PARTNERS

Health Department
Code or Building Inspection Agency
Property Owners

CRITICAL ELEMENTS

Staff requirements: Up to 1 FTE will be required for this strategy.

Other resource requirements: Accredited trainers and risk assessment training materials are required for preparing risk assessors; EPA's curriculum prepares lead sampling technicians.

Institutional capacity required: This strategy requires accredited risk assessment training programs with experienced instructors.

Cost considerations: Because risk assessment training is expensive, this strategy, especially if implemented on a large scale, can be costly. In some states, workforce development programs could be a possible source of funding. It may also be preferable for organizations to implement this strategy on a small scale. Lead sampling technician training is less costly and time-consuming, although trainees will be qualified to perform a more limited scope of testing.

Timing issues: After initial organization and scheduling, this strategy can be implemented at any time.

Feasibility of Implementation: High. This strategy should be feasible to implement.

POTENTIAL OBSTACLES/BARRIERS

Besides possible funding concerns, the only minor barrier to this strategy would be a lack of interest among property owners in training to check for hazards.

ADDITIONAL RESOURCES
N/A

ILLUSTRATION OF STRATEGY IN PRACTICE

Indiana Department of Environmental Management launched a campaign titled 2000 Families with a goal to train 200 property owners as risk assessors who would then offer 20 free risk assessments each. The campaign reached its training goal, and 120 of the newly trained risk assessors remained active in the discipline.

Jurisdiction or Target Area: Indiana

Primary Actors: Indiana Department of Environmental Management (IDEM)

Secondary Actor(s): N/A

Staffing utilized: 2 FTE were required for the duration of the 2000 Families campaign.

Other resources utilized: Accredited training providers.

Factors essential to implementation: Funding ($350,000 total) and interest among property owners were two critical factors essential to the implementation of the campaign.

Limitations/challenges/problems encountered: There were some challenges involved in the campaign. Not all of the risk assessors remained active, and not all of them followed through by offering 20 free risk assessments to families who wanted them. The campaign also dealt with challenges of coordination with the state regulatory agency.

Magnitude of Impact/Potential Impact: 1,200 dwelling units received free risk assessments through the campaign.

Potential for replication: Moderate. Given sufficient interest and dedication among property owners in a state or multi-county region, this strategy does hold potential for replication. However, initial funding for training is needed.

Contact for Specific Information
Tammy Johnson
Indiana Dept. of Environmental Management
317-273-5628
tsjohnso@dem.state.in.us

References for additional information
N/A

TEACH CODE INSPECTORS ABOUT LEAD SAFETY THROUGH JOINT VISITS

DESCRIPTION OF THE STRATEGY

When a health department or a community-based organization makes joint visits with code inspectors, they can demonstrate methods to identify lead hazards. Such visits can motivate greater attention to lead safety, heighten awareness of and skill in identifying existing lead hazards, and prompt agencies to have their code inspectors trained as lead hazard inspectors or risk assessors. In jurisdictions where existing lead hazards are a violation of building and/or housing codes, joint visits and enhanced lead hazard assessment skills for code inspectors can lead to more thorough enforcement of the code.

BENEFITS

Immediate/Direct Results: Joint visits immediately raise lead hazard awareness among code inspectors and increase enforcement against property owners whose buildings contain lead hazards, leading to control or removal of those hazards.

Public Health Benefits: As code inspectors' attention to peeling paint and lead dust hazards increases, more property owners will be required to attend to lead hazards before a child is poisoned.

Other Indirect/Collateral Benefits: A joint visit strategy can help create cooperative working relationships between agencies and/or organizations that may not have worked together in the past, and these relationships can help further goals of greater compliance with housing codes and addressing other housing-related health hazards. As news of stepped-up enforcement spreads, other property owners may be motivated to address lead hazards to avoid enforcement penalties. In cases where enforcement actions are not necessary because lead hazards are not discovered, code inspectors and their "lead-expert" partners can develop good relationships with landlords, tenants, and homeowners by providing information about lead safety and lead-safe work practices.

SCOPE OF POTENTIAL IMPACT

City- or County-Wide   Neighborhood/Community

PRIMARY ACTORS	KEY PARTNERS
Health Department	Property Owners
Code or Building Inspection Agency	Tenants
Community-based Organizations	

CRITICAL ELEMENTS

Staff requirements: In most instances, no new staff will be needed.

Other resource requirements: This strategy will require some educational materials.

Institutional capacity required: Inspectors will need training on identifying lead hazards, or even be trained as lead inspectors or risk assessors. The partners with expertise in lead hazards may need training on code inspection techniques, the locality's housing and/or building codes, and other details specific to each jurisdiction.

Cost considerations: Costs to implement this strategy should be minimal. Limited costs would be incurred if code inspectors go on to be trained as lead sampling technicians or in lead-safe work practices.

Timing issues: The implementation timeline will depend on training schedules, as well as how quickly partners with expertise in lead hazards can be integrated into the code inspection process.

Feasibility of Implementation: High. Implementation of this strategy should be easy.

POTENTIAL OBSTACLES/BARRIERS

The main potential obstacle for realizing this strategy would be the unwillingness of code inspection agencies to participate in a joint visit strategy, as some agencies may be inflexible in their operations due, for example, to previous questions about the independence and objectivity of the inspection program. Another potential obstacle could be a perceived lack of need for joint visits or the unwillingness or inability to add another task to code inspectors' list of duties.

ADDITIONAL RESOURCES

N/A

ILLUSTRATION OF STRATEGY IN PRACTICE

When the Environmental Health Coalition, a community-based organization in San Diego County, presented the National City Building and Safety Department with hard data from EHC's lead sampling activities that showed the existence of significant lead hazards, the Department decided that code inspectors needed more information about lead safety and how to identify lead hazards. At the same time, EHC's health promoters (*Promotoras*) wanted a better understanding of the code enforcement process.

The Department crafted the Community Housing Inspection Project, funded by a grant from the California Department of Housing and Community Development, to create a community code enforcement team consisting of code enforcement officers, a community relations health officer, property owners, and neighborhood residents and tenants. EHC's *Promotoras* cross-trained with code inspection and enforcement staff and then worked in joint inspection teams for one year in three target areas within the city.

Jurisdiction or Target Area: National City, CA

Primary Actors: Environmental Health Coalition (EHC) and the Building and Safety Department

Secondary Actor(s): N/A

Staffing utilized: Ten *Promotoras* participated in the cross-training; three National City code inspectors were trained on the basics of conducting a visual inspection to identify lead hazards.

Other resources utilized: Several code inspectors later sought training as risk assessors.

Factors essential to implementation: The cooperative attitude of the National City Building and Safety Department was critical to the implementation of this strategy. The dedication and interest from both the Promotoras and the code inspectors was also key.

Limitations/challenges/problems encountered: Language barriers were initially a challenge for this project, as most of the residents in the project's target area were Latino. EHC and the Department overcame these barriers by utilizing the *Promotoras'* translation skills. Another challenge for the project was the Department's reputation in the project's target area; prior to the project, the inspector for that portion of National City had severely alienated residents in those neighborhoods. The joint visits proved an excellent vehicle for building trust between the community and the Department.

Magnitude of Impact/Potential Impact: The cross training has allowed National City code inspectors and EHC's *Promotoras* to assess hundreds of properties for lead hazards so far. EHC's project also resulted in the Department adopting a protocol that empowers code inspectors to cite peeling paint as a nuisance in buildings constructed before 1979 and requires landlords to fix the hazard using lead-safe work practices.

Potential for replication: High. This strategy holds a good potential for replication in areas where significant lead hazards have been documented and where a cooperative attitude exists at the local code inspection agency.

Contacts for Specific Information

Letty Ayala
Environmental Health Coalition
619-235-0281
LeticiaA@environmentalhealth.org

Kathleen Trees
Director, Building and Safety Department
619-336-4210

References for additional information

1.   Environmental Health Coalition
         www.environmentalhealth.org

FINANCING AND SUBSIDIES

Access Electric Utility Public Benefit Funds

Create a Housing Trust Fund

Create a Special Real Estate Funding Mechanism

Deploy Enforcement Orders and Grant Incentives in Tandem

Establish a Revolving Fund to Stretch Dollars

Impose Fees on Real Estate Transactions and Related Professional Licenses

Impose Taxes or Fees on Polluters

Leverage CRA for Lead Safety and Healthy Homes

Make the Most of Fines and Penalties

Offer an Income Tax Credit for Abatement

Provide Local Property Tax Credits

Secure Dedicated Funding for Code Enforcement

ACCESS ELECTRIC UTILITY PUBLIC BENEFIT FUNDS

DESCRIPTION OF THE STRATEGY

Over the past decade, the deregulation of the electric utility industry has prompted the creation of public benefit funds in many states. The funds, which total more than $1.5 billion, support a wide range of activities related to energy conservation including home improvements that produce energy savings, such as increased insulation, air infiltration reduction, and sometimes window replacement. Policies are set by the state energy-related agency through negotiations with the key funding source(s).

Because such funds often target lower income households who suffer disproportionately from lead hazards the synergies are intriguing. The challenge is that these funds often strictly focus on energy and efforts to broaden the eligible activities could be perceived as diluting the programs' purpose. As a result, few utility benefits programs are currently factoring lead hazard reduction considerations into the program design.

BENEFITS

Immediate/Direct Results: Reducing lead hazards in the course of projects to make energy conservation improvements will have a direct impact on reducing lead exposure in high-risk properties. Such action can prevent lead poisoning and control lead hazards in the home.

Public Health Benefits: Repairing lead hazards through window replacement or repair and correction of moisture problems can reduce lead exposure and help to alleviate or prevent mold, which can exacerbate respiratory problems.

Other Indirect/Collateral Benefits: These actions can improve the overall building quality and energy usage (e.g., utility bills) making the building more durable and comfortable. Controlling lead hazards can also improve overall building quality, durability, and energy efficiency.

SCOPE OF POTENTIAL IMPACT

Statewide—Requires statewide commitment to make public benefit funds available for health and safety issues.

PRIMARY ACTORS	KEY PARTNERS
State Energy Agency	Housing Agency
Utilities	Community-based Organizations

CRITICAL ELEMENTS

Staff requirements: Short-term staff resources are required to develop the expansion of eligible activities to include lead and other health concerns. Staffing to clarify the actions that are eligible for public utility funding and appropriate protocols and procedures will need to be integrated into existing structures for the administration of public benefit funds.

Other resource requirements: Weatherization program crews may need additional training to check for and repair lead hazards.

Institutional capacity required: It is essential that the entity determining the scope and eligible activities for public benefit funds take steps to clarify that lead hazard control activities are eligible for funding. This may require a change in state statutory authority or a policy change by a state commission or entity that oversees the program and/or the utility that is providing the funds through the fee attached to utility bills.

Cost considerations: Once a decision is made to expand the use of the public benefits funds, the only cost of implementing the expansion is minimal staff to oversee the lead hazard repair services.

Timing issues: It may take over a year to gain policy agreement to expand the scope of activities funded by the public benefit funds to support lead hazard assessment and repair. If such actions are already eligible then an additional six months to one year is likely needed to get the program up and running.

Feasibility of Implementation: Moderate. Making public benefits funds available for lead hazard control work may require substantial advocacy and planning efforts.

POTENTIAL OBSTACLES/BARRIERS

A key potential obstacle may be opposition by energy conservation advocates who may be concerned that expanding the scope of eligible activities for funding by public benefit funds will reduce the number of homes receiving energy improvements.

ADDITIONAL RESOURCES

N/A

ILLUSTRATION OF THE STRATEGY IN PRACTICE

The New York State Energy Research and Development Authority (NYSERDA) administers programs funded by the System Benefits Charge (SBC) on the electricity transmitted and distributed by the state's investor-owned utilities. Originally, the fees for New York Energy $mart were intended to cover energy-related upgrades. Beginning in 2001, the program was expanded to address health concerns. This expansion required a policy decision at the state level to structure the supplemental health and safety component. The program covers up to 50% of the costs associated with energy-efficiency and indoor air quality improvements to a maximum of $5,000 for a single-family unit or $10,000 for a 2 - 4 family building. Low-interest loans are available for qualified applicants to cover the balance of the cost of the work. Total funds equal roughly $150 million per year for residential, commercial, and industrial properties combined; $40 million is invested in residential for both market and lower income.

Jurisdiction or Target Area: New York State

Primary Actor: New York State Energy Research and Development Authority (NYSERDA)

Secondary Actor(s): Building Performance Institute, Courtney Moriata, 518-899-2727, courtney@bpi.org.

Staffing utilized: Once agreement is reached on expansion of eligible activities to include health and safety concerns, the staff resources required to develop protocols and procedures to administer the program are nominal: overall, NYSERDA has one to two FTE working on the New York Energy $mart program.

Other resources utilized: NYSERDA contracted with a separate organization – Conservation Services Group (CSG) – to administer the program, audit energy and health results, process financial incentives, and manage loans. The Building Performance Institute (BPI) was engaged to develop work practice standards. A third entity with significant experience in adult education trains contractors (who are required to obtain training and certification to participate in the program). Contractors pay roughly $1,000 for each level of certification. NYSERDA reimburses the contractor for 75% of the training and certification fees.

Factors essential to implementation: Willing utility company and statewide administrator of public benefits funds, and motivated contractors who will pay for training/certification and absorb cost of lost work time to acquire credentials.

Limitations/challenges/problems encountered: Quality assurance is difficult. It is challenging to accurately report that the work occurred and determine if the work was performed consistent with program standards. CSG performs limited field inspections (roughly 15% overall) and BPI conducts sporadic field monitoring.

Magnitude of Impact/Potential Impact: In the initial three years of operation, approximately 4,000 homes have received energy upgrades. An unknown number have also received health upgrades to address combustion gases and possibly lead hazards. The average expenditure per unit is $7,500.

Potential for replication: Uncertain. NYSERDA is willing to share its experiences with other states (e.g., effective advertising strategies, standards, training curriculum, and program design materials). Key ingredients include: creating consumer demand for energy, comfort and health upgrades (where consumers are willing to pay for upgrades), varying marketing to target specific market segments, and developing standards to ensure consistent and quality work is performed. Realistic start up once there is agreement of funding is about two years to get the system working well.

Contacts for Specific Information

Rick Gerardi
Director Residential Programs
518-862-1090
reg@nyserda.org

Andrew Fisk
Senior Project Manager
518-862-1090
ajf@nyserda.org

References for additional information

1. NYSERDA web site with program details
    www.getenergysmart.org
2. Building Performance Institute
    www.bpi.org/

CREATE A HOUSING TRUST FUND

DESCRIPTION OF THE STRATEGY

Over 30 states and more than 250 local jurisdictions across the country have created housing trust funds to support affordable housing development. A housing trust fund is a distinct fund established by legislation, ordinance or resolution to receive public revenues that can only be spent on housing. Examples of dedicated revenues are real estate transfer taxes, document recording fees, new development fees, and proceeds from sale of publicly owned land. An administrative entity (such as an affordable housing commission, housing department, or housing finance agency) issues requests for proposals and awards funds according to priorities and goals established by the administering agency or the authorizing legislation. Most funds support both new construction and rehabilitation to benefit very low-income households and special needs populations. Most lead hazard control measures that improve a home's structure or surfaces qualify as eligible housing rehabilitation activities. The use of lead-safe work practices (LSWP) can be incorporated into program requirements.

BENEFITS

Immediate/Direct Results: Funds are available to increase the supply of lead-safe housing through the rehabilitation of substandard older properties (resulting in the elimination of lead hazards) and the construction of new housing.

Public Health Benefits: Creating decent affordable housing will prevent exposure to lead hazards, especially if priority is given to projects serving very low-income families that are at high risk for childhood lead poisoning.

Other Indirect/Collateral Benefits: Access to decent housing that is affordable to very low-income households and special needs populations enhances the learning and earning potential of the family and improves its ability to pay for health care, child care, and other necessities.

SCOPE OF POTENTIAL IMPACT

Statewide   Regional (e.g. multi-county)
City- or County-Wide

PRIMARY ACTOR

Housing Agency
Community-based Organizations

KEY PARTNERS

Property Taxation Agency

CRITICAL ELEMENTS

Staff requirements: This will vary depending on the size of the fund and the nature of the activities to be carried out.

Other resource requirements: The heart of a housing trust fund is a reliable, dedicated source of funds. A certainty of funds helps maintain an ongoing program that can sustain a production pipeline and maximize other opportunities.

Institutional capacity required: A housing trust fund needs to be administered by an agency or organization that is familiar with soliciting, reviewing, awarding, and monitoring grants and/or loans for affordable housing programs. The administering entity also needs to work closely with community-based organizations that understand and can articulate the needs and capacity of the community.

Cost considerations: The size of housing trust funds range from less than $100,000 per year to many millions of dollars per year, depending on the size of the jurisdiction and other factors.

Timing issues: A housing trust fund can be established at any time.

Feasibility of Implementation: High. The growing number of housing trust funds attests to the feasibility of establishing such funds.

POTENTIAL OBSTACLES/BARRIERS

The greatest difficulty in getting started is mobilizing the support to convince a legislative body that such a fund is needed and that an ongoing allocation of funds is required to make the fund operate effectively. This requires establishing clear cut goals and objectives, creating a coalition of organizations and individuals to support creation of the fund, and identifying alternative funding sources.

ADDITIONAL RESOURCES

1. The Center for Community Change's Housing Trust Fund Project
   www.communitychange.org/issues/housing/trustfundproject/

ILLUSTRATION OF STRATEGY IN PRACTICE

In 2001, the Board of Aldermen for the City of St. Louis adopted an ordinance to create an Affordable Housing Trust Fund (AHTF). The ordinance established an eleven-member St. Louis Affordable Housing Commission appointed by the Mayor and representing different interests throughout the City. The revenue source is a 2.625% sales tax on out-of-state purchases over $2,000. Loans and grants are authorized for the rehabilitation, modification, construction, and preservation of affordable and accessible housing. Grants are also authorized for accessibility modifications, lead-based paint abatement, and emergency assistance for home repairs and to prevent homelessness, transitional housing, and other similar uses.

Jurisdiction or Target Area: St. Louis, Missouri

Primary Actor: Affordable Housing Commission

Secondary Actor(s): N/A

Staffing Utilized: 0.5 FTE

Other resources utilized: N/A

Factors essential to implementation: A supplemental sales tax on out-of-state purchases is easy for jurisdictions in Missouri to administer because mechanisms already exist to collect use taxes at the state, county, and city level.

Limitations/problems encountered: Obtaining consensus of all the political leaders was difficult and time consuming.

Magnitude of Impact/Potential Impact: The St. Louis Affordable Housing Trust Fund has approximately $5 million available each year. The Fund provided a $100,000 grant to the St. Louis Lead Prevention Coalition to conduct lead abatement activities and program grants for housing-related services as well as "funds of last resort" to support the creation of 360 units during fiscal years 2002 and 2003.

Potential for replication: High.

Contact for Specific Information

Angela Conley
Executive Director
St. Louis Affordable Housing Commission
314-622-3400 Ext. 329

References for additional information

1. The St. Louis Affordable Housing Commission
   http://stlouis.missouri.org/affordablehousingcommission/

CREATE A SPECIAL REAL ESTATE FUNDING MECHANISM

DESCRIPTION OF THE STRATEGY

Funding for local or regional lead poisoning prevention activities can be generated through the addition of a fixed fee to the annual property tax bills for each dwelling unit in pre-1978 residential properties. The fee can be applied to all properties in the jurisdiction or only in those areas (e.g. some municipalities within a county) that opt to participate so that they can benefit from the resultant programs. The proceeds from assessing the fee can provide substantial start-up and/or supplementary funds for lead poisoning prevention programs.

BENEFITS

Immediate/Direct Results: A recurring source of funds is available to support primary prevention activities initiated by a local lead poisoning prevention program that cannot be financed through other mechanisms. The activities supported can include free training in lead safe work practices, screening of homes for lead hazards, and lead-safe painting supplies.

Public Health Benefits: Program interventions can be targeted to meet emerging needs and new opportunities at the local level, complementing federally funded blood lead screening and lead hazard control activities.

Other Indirect/Collateral Benefits: The owners of pre-1978 properties are reminded annually that their properties may have lead hazards and that there's a program that can help.

SCOPE OF POTENTIAL IMPACT

Statewide   Regional (e.g. multi-county)
City- or County-Wide

PRIMARY ACTORS

Property Taxation Agency

KEY PARTNERS

Health Department
Housing Agency
Human Services Agency
Community-based Organizations

CRITICAL ELEMENTS

Staff requirements: The tax agency staff must perform minor administrative activities at start-up, such as the modification of the property tax information system. No ongoing additional staffing is needed to implement the fee.

Other resource requirements: Tax agency must have the dates of construction for all residential real estate in the jurisdiction and the capacity to integrate the fee into the bills. If available, funds to print explanatory information to be included as an insert in the tax bill could optimize the benefit.

Institutional capacity required: It requires tax assessment authority and the enactment of a decision (e.g., via statute, ordinance, referendum) to add it to the code. The procedures for establishing property fees vary by location.

Cost considerations: There is no cost after start-up to the government agency responsible for tax collection. Although some landlords will pass the additional fee onto their renters by slightly increasing the rent, a small fee will have no substantial impact on housing affordability for owner-occupants or tenants.

Timing issues: Legislatures' meeting schedules (and electoral calendars in places where a referendum would be required) will determine when it is possible to enact policy to levy fees.

Feasibility of Implementation: Moderate. Political will, bolstered by the support of some residential property owners, is key to the implementation of a special real estate assessment mechanism, since a vote by either a legislative body and/or the electorate will be required to implement a new tax or other property-based tax. It should be possible to reach agreement to pursue the strategy in numerous jurisdictions, especially where there is concern about the problem of lead poisoning but action is more likely on approaches that require no new funds, staff, or equipment.

POTENTIAL OBSTACLES/BARRIERS

Lack of political will is the most significant potential barrier to establishing a special real estate assessment mechanism. In jurisdictions where a referendum is required for revenue-generating measures, the absence of widespread popular support may be a severe obstacle.

ADDITIONAL RESOURCES

N/A

ILLUSTRATION OF STRATEGY IN PRACTICE

The Alameda County Lead Poisoning Prevention Program (ACLPPP) is funded by a property-related fee established to address the sources of lead poisoning in the "County Service Area" (CSA), which consists of the four Alameda County cities where the city council has adopted an optional fee. The tax agency collects $10 per dwelling unit located in residential property built before 1978. The Joint Powers Authority Board of Directors, which is comprised of one representative from the city council of each of the four participating cities, one at-large community representative, and one representative of the County Board of Supervisors, oversees the funds and the functioning of the ACLPPP. Lead hazard evaluation and consultation services, training, painting preparation kits, and HEPA vacuum loans are provided to property owners in the participating cities. The program, a division of the Alameda County Community Development Agency, is also accountable to the County Board of Supervisors.

Jurisdiction or Target Area: Alameda County, CA (Oakland, Berkeley, Alameda, Emeryville)

Primary Actor: Alameda County Service Area, Joint Powers Authority, and Alameda County Lead Poisoning Prevention Program

Secondary Actor(s): N/A

Staffing utilized: Administration of the fee does not require staffing.

Other resources utilized: N/A

Factors essential to implementation: The program (ACLPPP) was established in 1991 as a result of an organized community effort led by People United for a Better Oakland (PUEBLO) to respond to a state Department of Health study that showed high levels of lead in Oakland's housing and in children's blood. PUEBLO simultaneously built public support for the creation of a county lead program and worked with county and city officials to establish the fee structure.

Limitations/problems encountered: None.

Magnitude of Impact/Potential Impact: This local funding source provided initial funding for the multi-disciplinary lead poisoning prevention program and therefore positioned the county to receive state funds for EBL case management as well as funds from the HUD Office of Healthy Homes and Lead Hazard Control. CSA funds support primary prevention activities while state funds support the case management of lead poisoned children and efforts to increase screening and HUD funds have supported lead hazard remediation.

Potential for replication: Moderate

Contact for Specific Information
Steve Schwartzberg
Deputy Director, CDA
510-567-8252

References for additional information
1. www.aclppp.org/alameda.shtml

DEPLOY ENFORCEMENT ORDERS
AND GRANT INCENTIVES IN TANDEM

DESCRIPTION OF THE STRATEGY

Public financing for the abatement of lead hazards, combined with code enforcement, provides both the carrot and the stick to provide lead-safe housing in high-risk neighborhoods. Landlords are most likely to be "persuaded" to address lead hazards if financial assistance is available to offset at least part of the cost of repairing/replacing windows and other lead hazards. The threat of being taken to court can be a powerful incentive to landlords. Combining code enforcement with financial incentives is especially useful to motivate action by landlords who own multiple high-risk properties and have limited resources.

BENEFITS

Immediate/Direct Results: Rental units are rendered safe from lead hazards. Depending on the scope of the program, results can range from a few units to an entire neighborhood or neighborhoods.

Public Health Benefits: Reduction in childhood lead poisoning. In addition, there is a heightened awareness of childhood lead poisoning and how to prevent it.

Other Indirect/Collateral Benefits: An improved standard of habitability: for example, windows that were dilapidated or painted shut become operable.

SCOPE OF POTENTIAL IMPACT

City- or County-Wide   Neighborhood/Community
Specific (Targeted) Population—Families with young children

PRIMARY ACTORS

Health Department
Community-based Organizations

KEY PARTNERS

City/County Prosecutors
Property Owners
Contractors

CRITICAL ELEMENTS

Staff requirements: Staff requirements will vary depending on the scope of the program and the extent to which activities are performed in-house or contracted out. Post-work clearance must be performed by a trained staff member or contractor who is certified.

Other resource requirements: A good database is critical to efficient operation. Access to standard professional specifications for the scope of work as well as uniform and reliable cost estimates for typical work will help build support from owners and landlords to participate in the program. In addition, for abatement programs, there must be a sufficient supply of trained and qualified contractors.

Institutional capacity required: There must be clear legal authority to require owners to correct lead hazards or at least to repair deteriorated paint. In addition, there must be an institutional structure that can enforce code violations. This may be a municipal court or an administrative hearing process that has enforcement authority.

Cost considerations: There must be a funding source to support lead hazard control as well as the code enforcement effort.

Timing issues: None; the program can be initiated at any time.

Feasibility of Implementation: Moderate. Can be implemented wherever the basic requirements are in place: political support, a staff commitment to working with landlords, legal authority, an operating code enforcement program, a skilled workforce, and financial aid to owners.

POTENTIAL OBSTACLES/BARRIERS

There must be political support to undertake the program and political will to use code enforcement authority to take action against recalcitrant landlords if they don't agree to repair their properties. Landlords can be expected to appeal to political leadership to forego or curtail the program.

Most difficult of all is getting landlords to buy in to the program. First, it is often difficult to find out who the actual owner of a specific property is. Second, it is even more difficult to get owners to come to a public meeting or agree to a private meeting. Third, if the owner does attend, he or she needs to be convinced to participate in the program and to pay for at least a portion of the repairs. The absence of a strategy on how to deal with landlords, including absentee landlords, can constitute a considerable barrier to success.

ADDITIONAL RESOURCES
N/A

ILLUSTRATION OF STRATEGY IN PRACTICE

The City of Milwaukee created the Milwaukee Pilot Ordinance to eliminate all lead hazards in pre-1950 homes in two high-risk neighborhoods. All rental property owners were required to register their properties in the program. For each property, the Health Department conducted a risk assessment and documented the scope of work needed. The City funded the repair of windows (or, rarely, their replacement); the owners were responsible for all other work required by the risk assessments. The City used certified workers for window repairs; the owners could do the other work themselves. All properties passed City-administered clearance examinations upon completion of the work and received certificates of lead safety.

Jurisdiction or Target Area: Milwaukee

Primary Actor: Milwaukee Health Department, Childhood Lead Poisoning Prevention Program

Secondary Actor(s): N/A

Staffing utilized: 0.5 FTE

Other resources utilized: N/A

Factors essential to implementation: City Council support was essential. The Council received input from the landlords who saw the pilot ordinance as better than strictly code enforcement. The support of community organizations and community residents was also critical. Funding from a HUD Lead Hazard Control grant covered the window repair work. A skilled workforce was developed to handle the high volume of repairs.

Limitations/problems encountered: Finding the owners/landlords was often very difficult. Getting them to "apply" for a risk assessment was even harder. City staff did mailings to owners and held group and individual meetings. The combination of hard sales in tandem with the threat of code enforcement was needed to win over reluctant landlords, especially since the amount available for window repairs was limited to approximately $2,000 per unit.

Magnitude of Impact/Potential Impact: Lead hazard control was completed in 800 units in one year. The owners of approximately 50 units were taken through the court system.

Potential for replication: High. The strategy can be replicated wherever there is a strong commitment from political leadership and staff to work with reluctant landlords and take them to court if necessary.

Contact for Specific Information
Richard Gaeta
Lead Hazard Prevention Manager
414-286-5788
rgaeta@milwaukee.gov

References for additional information
1. www.city.milwaukee.gov/display/router.asp?docid=2828

ESTABLISH A REVOLVING FUND TO STRETCH DOLLARS

DESCRIPTION OF THE STRATEGY

Instead of making outright grants of funds for lead hazard control projects, jurisdictions can make loans through a revolving loan fund that recycles the original pool of funds. Loans can be amortized or repayment deferred until the property is sold or refinanced. Financing terms can be indexed according to income so that the lowest income homeowners can access funds at very low and even no interest. Permanent revolving funds can be capitalized using an appropriation from the jurisdiction's general fund, a federal grant, or designating the receipts from a specific tax or fee, so that such monies are continuously reserved for a specified purpose.

BENEFITS

Immediate/Direct Results: Lead hazards are controlled, and the property is cleared by certified personnel.
Public Health Benefits: Reduction in lead-poisoned children.
Other Indirect/Collateral Benefits: The unit is safe for future occupants.

SCOPE OF POTENTIAL IMPACT

Statewide   City- or County-Wide

PRIMARY ACTORS
Housing Agency
Banks/Lending Institutions

KEY PARTNERS
Community-based Organizations
Property Owners

CRITICAL ELEMENTS

Staff requirements: One full-time person in the assigned agency is needed to set up the program. This includes developing program procedures and guidelines, preparing marketing materials, and establishing agreements with program partners such as health departments, lenders, and community-based organizations. A key policy issue is whether the agency administering the loan fund will manage the program or rely on other partners (banks, community-based nonprofit organizations, etc.) to perform outreach, prepare and process applications, and service the loans. If all work is done in-house, the staffing requirements will vary substantially depending on the volume of loans and the way the program is designed.

Other resource requirements: Program brochures, manuals, operating procedures for lending programs.

Institutional capacity required: There needs to be institutional capacity to make and/or service real estate loans, including knowledge of the industry and experience with lending programs. Ideally, the program is managed by a housing agency that has a track record with other financing mechanisms. Legislative authority and appropriations must create and fund the program; authority to use repayments for additional loans distinguishes revolving funds from one-time appropriations. Capacity to assist owners with applications is important and can be provided by community-based nonprofit organizations, city/county/state staff, or lenders.

Cost considerations: A revolving fund must initially be capitalized by designated funds. Annual or regular additions to the fund may be critical to create stability, meet growing demand, and assure continuation of the fund. Fees to process and service the loan and the cost of outreach need to be factored into the plan.

Timing issues: A revolving loan fund can be established at any time.

Feasibility of Implementation: Excellent if the institutional capacity is in place.

POTENTIAL OBSTACLES/BARRIERS

Making loans to low-income owners and/or investors in property rented to low-income families is often not a profitable venture. Financial institutions are experienced and efficient in processing loans; however, a bank will probably need an incentive such as a fee unless it is willing to do the work to maintain or improve its Community Reinvestment Act (CRA) rating.

Capacity must also be established to get referrals or generate applications, assist owners with the application process, qualify applicants, and prepare complete applications for whomever processes the application. A state or local agency may be well served by relying on community-based organizations (CBOs) to reach and encourage applications from the owners of highest risk properties.

ADDITIONAL RESOURCES

N/A

ILLUSTRATION OF STRATEGY IN PRACTICE

MassHousing provides financing to owners of one- to four-unit properties to abate lead-based paint. Low-income owner-occupants are eligible for loans with 0 percent interest for which payment is not due until the property's sale or refinancing. Nonprofit organizations and "investor-owners" (landlords who do not live in a unit in the property) that own properties that are being rented to income eligible households are eligible for loans that must be repaid in the near term. The maximum loan amounts are: Single-family—$20,000; 2-family—$25,000; 3-family—$30,000; and 4-family—$35,000.

Applications are made through local housing rehabilitation agencies (LRAs). Completed applications are processed and underwritten by Fleet National Bank. Both the LRA and the bank receive fees. The bank sells the loans to MassHousing which services the loan. Many of the loans originate from court orders resulting from an inspection triggered by the identification of a child with an elevated blood lead level.

Jurisdiction or Target Area: Massachusetts

Primary Actor: MassHousing (Massachusetts Housing Finance Agency)

Secondary Actor: N/A

Staffing utilized: 1 FTE

Other resources utilized: N/A

Factors essential to implementation: There needs to be continuous funding from the State, and authority to reuse repayments. Massachusetts has a strong statewide network of nonprofit housing organizations to assist homeowners in preparing applications.

Limitations/problems encountered: Massachusetts found that bond funds didn't work well; a State appropriation was much better. The borrower needs to be current on the mortgage, taxes, and utilities.

Magnitude of Impact/Potential Impact: Approximately 200 – 300 loans are made each year. Nearly $50 million has been loaned since 1997.

Potential for replication: Very high. There must be a nonprofit network or other means to assist owners in applying and, if the MassHousing model is followed, a bank willing to participate.

Contacts for Specific Information

Virginia Healy-Kenney
Manager, Home Ownership Production
MassHousing
617-854-1326
vhealykenney@masshousing.com

Rose Hughes
Underwriter
Fleet National Bank
860-409-5892
rose_a_hughes@fleet.com

References for additional information

1. MassHousing
   www.masshousing.com. Click on Get the Lead Out.

IMPOSE FEES ON REAL ESTATE TRANSACTIONS AND RELATED PROFESSIONAL LICENSES

DESCRIPTION OF THE STRATEGY

Imposing fees on real estate transactions and on the licenses of professionals who procure housing, risk management, or lead services can help subsidize the cost of managing public sector systems for lead poisoning prevention. Fees levied on real estate transactions (e.g. for the recording of deeds or tax stamps) and on licenses for professions and disciplines such as real estate agents, insurance agents, lead inspectors, risk assessors, lead abatement contractors, and others can be a source of dedicated income for lead poisoning prevention programs. These types of strategies would be more common at the state level, but enactment and implementation is possible at the county and municipal levels as well.

BENEFITS

Immediate/Direct Results: New or increased recurring funding sources are immediately created as the fee structure goes into effect. These funds can be used to support primary prevention programs that may have little, if any, funding from other sources.

Public Health Benefits: Funds from these fees or surcharges can be used to fund existing childhood lead poisoning prevention programs as well as initiatives that complement efforts already in existence.

Other Indirect/Collateral Benefits: By targeting home purchases and individuals directly involved with buying, selling, and insuring housing, such fees could raise awareness among homebuyers, real estate agents, mortgage lenders, insurers, and others about lead poisoning prevention issues. Such a strategy may also reinforce the responsibility of buyers, agents, and others to ensure that the home involved in a specific transaction is lead-safe.

SCOPE OF POTENTIAL IMPACT

Statewide   City- or County-Wide

PRIMARY ACTORS

State Licensing and Certification Agencies

KEY PARTNERS

Code or Building Inspection Agency
Housing Agency
Property Owners
Certified Lead Abatement Contractors
Insurance companies and brokers

CRITICAL ELEMENTS

Staff requirements: Minor to moderate administrative activities would be required at the start-up of a strategy that imposes a fee on real estate transactions or a surcharge on certain professional licenses. It is unlikely that any new staff would be required to implement such fees or surcharges.

Other resource requirements: In the case of professional license surcharges, the agency(s) that oversee the licensing may need to be involved in administering the strategy.

Institutional capacity required: New statutory or code sections, naming the specific real estate transactions or professional licenses involved, must be added, and the agency(s) involved may need to promulgate new regulations to implement the strategy.

Cost considerations: Small start-up costs to the government agencies responsible for the collection of the new fees or surcharges can be expected, but no further costs should exist beyond this transition period.

Timing issues: None

Feasibility of Implementation: Moderate. Political will, bolstered by the support of individuals, community and statewide organizations, and those who have been adversely affected by lead poisoning will be key to implementing this strategy. Partnering with professionals in the real estate or insurance worlds who are concerned about or aware of lead hazards in homes would also be useful.

POTENTIAL OBSTACLES/BARRIERS

The lack of political will to impose a new fee or surcharge is the major obstacle that could block the realization of this strategy. Once put in place, a license surcharge strategy may have to overcome overburdened licensing agencies or inefficient transfer of revenues. A minimal fee on real estate transactions is not likely to face significant implementation barriers.

ADDITIONAL RESOURCES

N/A

ILLUSTRATION OF STRATEGY IN PRACTICE

In Massachusetts, surcharges are imposed on the annual fees of a variety of professional licenses. These surcharges are imposed on individuals licensed as real estate brokers and property and casualty insurance agents, as well as on mortgage brokers, mortgage lenders, small loan agencies, and individuals licensed to perform lead inspections. The surcharge is generally $25 per license or renewal, though mortgage brokers, lenders, and small loan agencies pay a $100 surcharge.

The strategy was enacted by the state in 1993 to provide additional funds to the Childhood Lead Poisoning Prevention Program. Amounts raised by the surcharges are deposited into a retained revenue account, known as the Lead Paint Education and Training Trust Account, for use by the Department of Health in lead poisoning prevention activities, including primary prevention efforts.

Jurisdiction or Target Area: Massachusetts

Primary Actors: Dept. of Public Health, Childhood Lead Poisoning Prevention Program; Dept. of Labor and Industries; Div. of Professional Licensure; Div. of Banks; Div. of Insurance.

Secondary Actor(s): Div. of Professional Licensure; Dept. of Labor and Industries; Div. of Banks; Div. of Insurance.

Staffing utilized: 0.5 FTE.

Other resources utilized: N/A

Factors essential to implementation: The cooperation of professionals impacted by this strategy is key, as is the level of priority each licensing board places on collecting the surcharges. Two additional factors are essential to the continuing implementation of this strategy:
1. The continued existence of the statutory authority contained in the Acts of 1993; and
2. The timely distribution of the surcharges to the Trust Account for disbursement to DPH

Limitations/challenges/problems encountered: There have been no major challenges in implementing the surcharge strategy. However, the Office of the State Auditor found that some professions were not being billed for the surcharge in a timely manner in 2000; the responsible agency subsequently corrected the problem, and in 2002, the Legislature mandated that it collect the surcharge in direct connection with the license renewal process.

IMPOSE FEES ON REAL ESTATE TRANSACTIONS AND RELATED PROFESSIONAL LICENSES

Magnitude of Impact/Potential Impact: The surcharge strategy raises about $1.25 million per year for DPH/CLPPP. This gives the department and the program much needed funds to engage in a variety of childhood lead poisoning prevention activities.

Potential for replication: Moderate. In states with sufficient political will, fee-based funding strategies, such as surcharges on specific professional licenses, could be readily replicated.

Contacts for Specific Information

Paul Hunter
Director
Childhood Lead Poisoning Prevention Program
617-624-5757
paul.hunter@state.ma.us

Mary Madden
Supervisor
Agent & Broker Licensing, Division of Insurance
617-521-7794
Mary.Madden@state.ma.us

References for additional information

1. Mass. Acts of 1993, Chapter 482, Section 22
2. Mass. Childhood Lead Poisoning Prevention Program
   www.state.ma.us/dph/clppp/clppp.htm

IMPOSE TAXES OR FEES ON POLLUTERS

DESCRIPTION OF THE STRATEGY

States and local jurisdictions that have appropriate authority can impose taxes and/or fees on corporations that are judged responsible for contributing to the existence of an environmental health or pollution problem, including those companies that have contributed to the existence of lead hazards in housing. The revenue from these taxes and fees can be used to fund primary prevention programs.

BENEFITS

Immediate/Direct Results: New or increased funding sources are immediately created as the tax or fee structure goes into effect. These funds can be channeled into a variety of primary prevention efforts that may not have other sources of sustained funding.

Public Health Benefits: Funds from these taxes or fees can be used to fund either already existing public health programs related to the prevention of childhood lead poisoning, or possibly expand primary prevention efforts to reach a greater number of people.

Other Indirect/Collateral Benefits: By targeting corporations that are responsible for the production of goods that caused indoor lead contamination, a tax or fee on these polluters helps shift the burden away from taxpayers and individuals who are impacted by environmental health hazards.

SCOPE OF POTENTIAL IMPACT

Statewide

City- or County-Wide

Regional (e.g. multi-county)

Neighborhood/Community

PRIMARY ACTORS

Health Department

State Taxing Authority

KEY PARTNERS

Community-based Organizations

Political Affiliates

CRITICAL ELEMENTS

Staff requirements: Minor to moderate administrative activities would be required at the start-up of a new tax or fee on polluters. It is unlikely that any new staffing would be required.

Other resource requirements: The taxing agency must have all information pertaining to the specific corporations or class of corporations upon which the new tax or fee is to be imposed.

Institutional capacity required: A new statutory or code section, naming the specific corporation or class of corporations to be targeted with the new tax or fee, must be added. In many states, taxing authority of this nature must be approved on the state level before being implemented by local jurisdictions.

Cost considerations: Small start-up costs to the government agency responsible for the collection of the new tax or fee can be expected, but no further costs should exist beyond this transition period. Costs to targeted corporations will likely be passed onto to retailers, and in turn, to consumers.

Timing issues: Because new statutory authority may be needed to implement taxes or fees on polluters, the implementation of the strategy will depend on legislative calendars, committee hearing schedules, and local government meeting schedules. In some areas, some taxes and fees carry "sunset" provisions, meaning they must be reviewed and reauthorized on a periodic basis. In other areas, tax or fee structure changes such as this are permanent.

Feasibility of Implementation: Moderate. Political will, bolstered by the support of consumers, community and statewide organizations, and those who have been adversely affected are key to the success of efforts to impose taxes and fees on polluters. Some may be opposed to imposing taxes or fees on selected corporations because that might be seen as "bad for the general business climate" in the state or local area. Others may support shifting the burden of financially supporting lead poisoning prevention programs to those directly responsible for indoor environmental health problems caused by lead.

POTENTIAL OBSTACLES/BARRIERS

The lack of political will to impose a new tax or fee, especially on powerful corporate interests, is the major obstacle that could block the realization of this strategy. Many states and local areas have very strong business lobbies, and targeted corporations themselves may be willing to spend large amounts of time and money to defeat a strategy that would increase their overall costs.

ADDITIONAL RESOURCES

N/A

ILLUSTRATION OF STRATEGY IN PRACTICE

The Childhood Lead Poisoning Prevention Act was passed in California in 1991. The state act provides funds for county programs to identify children at risk for lead poisoning and to work toward reducing children's exposure to lead hazards.

The program implemented under the act is funded by a fee imposed on corporations that previously, or currently, bear responsibility for the production and sale of lead or products containing lead. This fee also extends to corporations and businesses that are responsible for other sources of lead or that have contributed or continue to significantly contribute to environmental lead contamination (indoor and outdoor). The fee is assessed on each individual corporation based on two criteria:

- The corporation's past and present responsibility for environmental lead contamination
- The corporation's "market share" responsibility for environmental lead contamination

The two criteria allow for greater fees to be imposed on those corporations that hold a greater responsibility for environmental lead contamination.

Jurisdiction or Target Area: California

Primary Actors: California State Board of Equalization; California State Department of Health Services/ California Childhood Lead Poisoning Prevention Branch

Secondary Actor(s): N/A

Staffing utilized: No information provided.

Other resources utilized: N/A

Factors essential to implementation: Factors important to the initial implementation of the tax on polluters included the political will to hold polluters financially responsible for their actions, as well as the efforts of community and environmental groups throughout the state. The factor essential to the continuing implementation of the fee is the continued existence of the statutory authority in the California Health and Safety Code

Limitations/challenges/problems encountered: None identified.

Magnitude of Impact/Potential Impact: Annually, $12 million is collected for county programs in California via this fee. The impact is significant in that the fees are the main source of funds for the state's Childhood Lead Poisoning Prevention Program and the county-based programs.

Potential for replication: Moderate. In states and localities where the political will is present, fee-based funding strategies such as this could be readily replicated with a minimal use of resources.

Contacts for Specific Information

Larrie Lance
Chief, Lead Hazard Reduction Section
Childhood Lead Poisoning Prevention Branch
510-622-5000

Jerri Dale
Chief, Customer and Taxpayer Services Division
State Tax Equalization Board
916-445-6188

References for additional information

1. California Health and Safety Code Sections 105275-105310
   www.leginfo.ca.gov/cgi-bin/displaycode?section=hsc&group=105001-106000&file=105275-105310
2. California Lead Poisoning Prevention Branch
   www.dhs.ca.gov/childlead/
3. State Tax Equalization Board
   www.boe.ca.gov/sptaxprog/occupleadfee.htm

LEVERAGE COMMUNITY REINVESTMENT ACT FOR LEAD SAFETY AND HEALTHY HOMES

DESCRIPTION OF THE STRATEGY

The federal Community Reinvestment Act (CRA) was enacted in 1977 to challenge widespread discrimination in mortgage lending and encourage banks to help meet the credit needs of all segments of their communities, including low- and moderate-income neighborhoods. Banks may provide loans, grants, technical assistance or services to support community development activities that serve low- and moderate-income communities, including assistance with the cost of abating or controlling lead hazards in housing. Banks report relevant activity to their respective federal regulatory agencies which monitor the banks and issue public ratings of the banks' CRA activities in three areas: lending, investment, and services. These ratings affect whether regulators will permit banks to merge or expand. Many banks are therefore open to partnerships with local agencies or community-based organizations that are seeking financing or other support for specific proposals.

BENEFITS

Immediate/Direct Results: The loans and services result in housing rehabilitation or lead hazard control, or even education and outreach on preventing childhood lead poisoning

Public Health Benefits: Depending on the nature of the CRA investment, fewer children are exposed to lead-based paint hazards and/or the supply of lead-safe housing is increased.

Other Indirect/Collateral Benefits: Some financial institutions have established community lending programs with designated officers who work full time. Lending institutions that provide an ongoing point of contact can establish working relationships with public agencies and community-based organizations, sustain capacity-building, and become involved in a broad spectrum of activities.

SCOPE OF POTENTIAL IMPACT

Statewide
City- or County-Wide

Regional (e.g. multi-county)
Neighborhood/Community

PRIMARY ACTORS

Banks/Lending Institutions

KEY PARTNERS

Health Department
Housing Agency
Community-based Organizations

CRITICAL ELEMENTS

Staff requirements: Once a financial institution decides to increase lending or make qualified investments in underserved communities, it must develop appropriate agreements, policy guidelines, and operating procedures. Some banks execute contractual agreements with a nonprofit organization to administer the activity and assist in developing processing procedures for loans and establishing program eligibility criteria. These activities may require a significant investment of time and effort, depending on the experience level of and extent of initiative on the part of the lender and the nonprofit partner.

Other resource requirements: It is easiest for the bank to partner with an experienced nonprofit agency operating an effective program that needs added funding or assistance to expand into new areas or activities.

Institutional capacity required: The federal legal authority for CRA activity is already established (12 U.S.C. 2901).

Cost considerations: The modest cost of operating community lending activities, as an in-house service and/or under contract with a nonprofit partner, counts as a CRA service.

Timing issues: Can be implemented at any time.

Feasibility of Implementation: Moderate where there is a bank that is interested in undertaking CRA activity involving prevention of childhood lead poisoning.

POTENTIAL OBSTACLES/BARRIERS

The typical problem is finding or designing an activity or program that meets the bank's criteria for lending or investment and also provides substantive assistance. For instance, if the CRA activity is lending to abate or control lead hazards, the bank must be willing to discount its loans or make other changes to its lending guidelines to make the loans attractive to borrowers. A reduction of 1% in the interest rate will generally not be sufficient. Many potential borrowers will not have good credit ratings. A modest relaxation of credit standards may qualify a few borrowers that otherwise could not borrow at conventional lending rates. However, it will probably be necessary to supplement lending at below-market rates with grants for a portion of the cost.

ADDITIONAL RESOURCES

1. Federal Financial Institutions Examination Council
   www.ffiec.gov
2. National Community Reinvestment Coalition
   www.ncrc.org

ILLUSTRATION OF STRATEGY IN PRACTICE

Mahoning County has a contract with First Place Bank to provide financing for lead hazard control in rental properties. Potential borrowers are referred to the bank which qualifies the borrowers. The County then conducts an inspection/risk assessment and prepares a scope of work and a cost estimate. The bank underwrites the loan but writes off the closing costs, which average about $1,700 per loan. The County buys down 50% of the loan up to $12,500 (County maximum: $6,250); the borrower pays 100 percent of the loan amount over $12,500. The owner hires a licensed contractor to perform the work. The County pays any relocation costs and clears the property to ensure that lead dust hazards are not left behind. First Place Bank receives CRA credit for the closing costs that it pays.

Jurisdiction or Target Area: Mahoning County, Ohio

Primary Actors: Mahoning County Lead Hazard Control Program and First Place Bank

Secondary Actor(s): N/A

Staffing utilized: 0.25 FTE

Other resources utilized: N/A

Factors essential to implementation: The primary factor is a bank willing to participate; i.e., absorb the closing costs in exchange for CRA credits. Secondly, there must be willing landlords who see the remediation of lead hazards as in their interest.

Limitations/problems encountered: The biggest problem is getting landlords to participate. They must become part of the solution.

Magnitude of Impact/Potential Impact: Borrowing by owners of rental property is made feasible by two factors: The cost of borrowing is reduced when the bank waives closing costs, and the cost or rehab is partially offset by a grant from the County of up to $6,250. Approximately 40 – 50 units will be completed with funds from a HUD Lead Hazard Control grant and the First Place Bank subsidy.

Potential for replication: This can be replicated in communities with a bank willing to make concessions in their lending in return for CRA credits.

Contacts for Specific Information

Gary Singer
Director
Mahoning County Lead Hazard Control Program
330-740-2130 ext 7172
gsinger@mahoningcounty.org

Rocky Page
Vice President, Mortgage Lending
First Place Bank
330-726-3396 ext 1150
rpage@fpfc.net

References for additional information
N/A

MAKE THE MOST OF FINES AND PENALTIES

DESCRIPTION OF THE STRATEGY

Typically, fines and penalties that government agencies collect revert to the treasury's general fund. Designating a special fund, revolving or otherwise, offers a mechanism for such receipts to be reserved for a special purpose such as lead hazard control or promoting lead safe work practices. Rather than having all taxpayers fund code enforcement and other services that are directed toward a problem few, jurisdictions can charge violators fees to cover costs of inspection, investigation, and enforcement of building codes and other ordinances related to lead hazards and poisoning prevention.

BENEFITS

Immediate/Direct Results: This strategy allows municipalities, counties, and even states to fund important prevention programs and enforcement actions that may not receive adequate money from the general fund. The revenue generated from designated fines and penalties can then be used to support more code enforcement, training sessions on lead-safe work practices, lead hazard control, and other primary prevention measures.

Public Health Benefits: Presumably, with significant penalties in place for violating statutes or codes related to lead hazards, property owners will be apt to follow the rules, thus engaging in lead-safe work practices, reducing lead hazards in homes, and ultimately lowering the chance that children will be exposed to lead. The primary prevention measures funded by fines and penalties from those property owners who don't play by the rules will also reduce children's exposure to lead hazards.

Other Indirect/Collateral Benefits: As word spreads throughout the area affected by the possibility of fines or penalties (i.e. the city, county, or state), property owners, especially landlords, will become more aware of the issues surrounding lead poisoning in children, lead-safe work practices, and reducing and controlling lead hazards in homes.

SCOPE OF POTENTIAL IMPACT

Statewide	Regional (e.g. multi-county)
City- or County-Wide	Neighborhood/Community

PRIMARY ACTORS

Health Department
Code or Building Inspection Agency

KEY PARTNERS

Property Taxation Agency

CRITICAL ELEMENTS

Staff requirements: Since this income is generated by existing housing, building, and/or health code enforcement programs, no additional staff should be necessary.

Other resource requirements: Implementation would require systems for tracking data on fines and penalties generated from codes, as well as statutes governing lead hazards and lead safe work practices (or other building or housing provisions).

Institutional capacity required: Statutory and regulatory authority needed to create the specialized fund and designate the use of the fines and penalties. Code inspection and enforcement staff may need to be trained on how to recognize lead hazards and unsafe work practices if the jurisdiction has not previously focused on these areas.

Cost considerations: In almost all instances, no new enforcement agency or staff will be needed. One possible problem is that the cost of compliance as well as fines and penalties may be passed on to tenants; to mitigate this situation, consideration should be given to using some proceeds for targeted rent subsidies as needed.

Timing issues: Enforcement, the collection of fines and penalties, and the flow of money from the specialized fund will depend on the workload of the authorized agency.

Feasibility of Implementation: High. Local governments are always looking for revenue generators. Since this approach enables a program to be self-funded, holds bad actors accountable, and doesn't require a general tax increase, it should be quite feasible to implement.

POTENTIAL OBSTACLES/BARRIERS

Landlord associations will resist enactment and enforcement of code provisions for fines and penalties. Overburdened building inspection, housing, and health departments' implementation and enforcement may be lackluster, resulting in a low rate of collection of penalties.

ADDITIONAL RESOURCES

N/A

ILLUSTRATION OF STRATEGY IN PRACTICE

Chapter 34, Sec. 3407 of the San Francisco Building Code governs work practices used in the removal of exterior lead-based paint. In general, the removal of lead-based paint from exterior surfaces of buildings and structures in San Francisco is banned unless the person performing the work follows strict lead-safe work practices standards. Each year, property owners and contractors violate various provisions of the ordinance and are penalized accordingly. Any monetary penalties collected are funneled into a specialized Building Inspection Fund, which supports the department's various functions, including enforcement of the lead-based paint work standards for exterior surfaces.

Jurisdiction or Target Area: San Francisco, CA

Primary Actor: San Francisco Dept. of Building Inspection

Secondary Actor(s): N/A

Staffing utilized: The department utilizes staff on hand to implement and administer the specialized fund.

Other resources utilized: N/A

Factors essential to implementation: The main essential factor for implementation of this strategy in San Francisco is the cooperation between two sections of the Department of Building Inspection—the Lead Abatement Section and the Administration and Finance Section. Code enforcement and penalty collection officials rely on the City Tax Collector to collect delinquent penalties and on department hearing officers when a penalty is appealed. Underlying all of this is the code authority already in place.

Limitations/challenges/problems encountered: None listed.

Magnitude of Impact/Potential Impact: On average, the Building Inspection Fund receives between $1.2 and $1.7 million each year from fines and penalties. A portion of these funds is used to support the enforcement of lead-safe work practices standards for exterior surfaces. This is the major source of funding for this enforcement work; no general revenue is used for the enforcement of the work practices standards.

Potential for replication: The potential for replication of this approach to the fines and penalties strategy is high. It is relatively easy to administer, and it is easily integrated into existing code enforcement and penalty structures.

Contacts for Specific Information

Louise Kimball
San Francisco Dept. of Building Inspection
Lead Abatement Section
415-558-6598

Taras Madison
San Francisco Dept. of Building Inspection
Administration and Finance Section
415-558-6239

References for additional information

1. City and County of San Francisco Building Code, 2001 Edition, Vol. 1, Chapter 34—Existing Structures, Sec. 3407 (specifically Sec. 3407.7)
2. City and County of San Francisco Dept. of Building Inspection
   www.sfgov.org/site/dbi_index.asp

OFFER AN INCOME TAX CREDIT FOR ABATEMENT

DESCRIPTION OF THE STRATEGY

One approach to funding lead hazard control outside of general fund appropriations is for governments to offer a credit on federal, state, or local income taxes to property owners who expend funds for eligible activities. A tax credit's advantage of extremely low administrative costs is balanced against the problem that tax credits are difficult to target and frequently provide little or no benefit for very low-income properties that generate little or no tax liability.

BENEFITS

Immediate/Direct Results: A tax credit is a way to finance the cost of lead hazard control, subject to cost limitations and other operational requirements such as the use of certified contractors. Although income tax credits provide dollar-for-dollar reduction in tax liability at the end of a tax year, up to the maximum amount specified, the funds are not available to pay for the cost of abatement at the time the work is performed.
Public Health Benefits: Additional lead-safe houses will expose fewer children to lead hazards.
Other Indirect/Collateral Benefits: Ease of administration.

SCOPE OF POTENTIAL IMPACT

Statewide   City- or County-Wide

PRIMARY ACTORS	KEY PARTNERS
Property Taxation Agency	Property Owners
	Contractors

CRITICAL ELEMENTS

Staff requirements: The staffing requirements to implement a tax credit for abatement are minimal. There is the initial need to draft regulations to incorporate the credit into a state's tax code as well as explanatory materials to foster general public understanding. Once the tax credit is implemented, it becomes just another line item on a tax return.

Other resource requirements: There must be a mechanism for verifying that a property for which a credit is claimed has lead hazards and that the work has addressed the lead hazards (through either abatement or interim controls), leaving the property or work area lead-safe at the end of the job. Jurisdictions should specify that the hazard control and hazard determination/clearance work be performed by appropriate trained or certified personnel. There must be a sufficient supply of qualified personnel available to property owners.

Institutional capacity required: A tax structure and administrative agency that can fairly administer a tax credit as part of an income tax system.

Cost considerations: It is very difficult to estimate the financial impact of a tax credit for lead paint abatement on a jurisdiction's tax revenue, since it is impossible to predict how many taxpayers will take advantage of this opportunity.

Timing issues: None.

Feasibility of Implementation: Extremely easy to implement, but difficult to enact when state and local revenues are constrained.

POTENTIAL OBSTACLES/BARRIERS

Successfully amending a complex tax code may be daunting for people and organizations normally dedicated to health and housing issues. The tax credit must be large enough to create an incentive for property owners to spend their own money for lead hazard control or abatement. At the same time, the cost must be reasonable enough that it can be borne by the state.

ADDITIONAL RESOURCES

1. Federal income tax credit legislation for lead abatement is now pending (S. 1228).

ILLUSTRATION OF STRATEGY IN PRACTICE

The Commonwealth of Massachusetts' "deleading " income tax credit, which has been in place since 1994, offers a model for other states interested in helping residents pay for the cost of abating lead hazards. The owner of a residential property can claim a tax credit equal to the lesser of the cost of deleading, or $1,500, for the containment or abatement of lead hazards, including the replacement of window units. A tax credit equal to the lesser of one-half of the cost of deleading, or $500, is available to offset the cost of bringing the property into interim compliance, using interim control measures, pending full compliance. Several steps are necessary to claim the credit: the property must be inspected by a licensed inspector; the property is then "deleaded" by a MA-licensed contractor; a licensed inspector issues a letter of compliance or a letter of interim control; and the owner files a copy of the inspector's letter with the owner's income tax return. The tax credit is a dollar-for-dollar offset for the actual amount spent against taxes owed. Any unused portion of the credit may be carried forward from the year that a credit was first claimed to any of the next seven years. Some activities may be undertaken by a "qualified unlicensed individual" pursuant to State regulations.

Jurisdiction or Target Area: Massachusetts

Primary Actor: Massachusetts Department of Revenue

Secondary Actor(s): N/A

Staffing utilized: No dedicated staff.

Other resources utilized: N/A

Factors essential to implementation: State legislation is the essential prerequisite. There is no staff dedicated to implementing or enforcing this particular element of the tax code.

Limitations/problems encountered: The relatively modest size of the tax credit ($1,500) limits the use of a tax credit as an incentive to undertake lead hazard abatement activities. Since most deleading projects in Massachusetts cost several thousand dollars, the tax credit is seldom the deciding factor in financing the cost of lead hazard remediation.

Magnitude of Impact/Potential Impact: The dollar impact on the State is not known.

Potential for replication: This can be implemented in any jurisdiction with an income tax and a legislature willing to create a tax credit for the purpose of abating lead hazards. The potential small loss of revenue will be weighed against other competing budgetary interests.

Contact for Specific Information

Massachusetts Department of Revenue
617-887-MDOR

References for additional information

1. See www.dor.state.ma.us/help/guides/abate_amend/personal/issues/leadpnt.htm for a summary of the lead paint removal credit.

PROVIDE LOCAL PROPERTY TAX CREDITS

DESCRIPTION OF THE STRATEGY

Local governments could offer a credit on or forgiveness of property taxes to property owners who make expenditures on specified activities such as window replacement, lead hazard control, or correction of other health and safety hazards—just as credits are provided currently in some locales for marginal properties that are substantially improved. A property tax credit could be very narrowly targeted, for example to a single high-risk neighborhood within designated boundaries. While property tax revenue reductions ultimately have the same budgetary impact as expenditure increases, some jurisdictions may find that tax credits are more palatable than increasing local agency budgets. No specific lead paint or health-related property tax credit exists anywhere today, although a bill (HB1039) to create a property tax credit for lead hazard reduction for residential and child care properties was introduced in Maryland in 2004.

BENEFITS

Immediate/Direct Results: Improvements related to lead safety and other health considerations are far more likely to be made by owners who can recoup some of their costs. Property tax credits provide more direct and immediate benefits to owners of low-income properties than income tax deductions or credits. Making the credit dependent upon independent verification of the work provides an opportunity to build in quality controls.
Public Health Benefits: Lead hazard reduction directly reduces lead exposure to children.
Other Indirect/Collateral Benefits: Improvements will generally increase property values and durability of housing, restore vacant buildings, provide employment opportunities, and increase community pride.

SCOPE OF POTENTIAL IMPACT

Statewide
City- or County-Wide
Neighborhood/Community—Credits could be narrowly targeted to highest-risk geographic areas
Specific (Targeted) Population—Credits could be targeted to rental housing only, or based on income of owners or occupants

PRIMARY ACTORS
Property Taxation Agency

KEY PARTNERS
Community-based Organizations
Property Owners
Tenants
Contractors
Homeowners

CRITICAL ELEMENTS

Staff requirements: Approximately 1.0 FTE might be needed to process applications and approve repairs for a program in a major jurisdiction. Other administrative aspects of this program probably could be carried out within the existing staffing and budget of any state or local revenue or property tax agency.

Other resource requirements: Some new administrative processes and forms would be needed.

Institutional capacity required: Changes in state, county, and local tax law may be necessary, depending on the jurisdiction.

Cost considerations: Losses in property tax revenue would be the main cost to a jurisdiction. There would be marginal administrative costs in ensuring that required repairs are actually done and auditing claims to avoid fraudulent use of the credit. Long-term enhancement of property value may partially offset the lost tax revenue as lead safety becomes valued in the marketplace. Collateral improvements to property condition (e.g., increased energy efficiency, new windows, plumbing and roof repairs) will increase property value and durability, which in turn should increase future property tax revenues and help arrest blight.

Timing issues: No seasonal or cyclical considerations other than the fact that policies that reduce tax revenue are more likely to succeed in times of budget surpluses. Timeline to implement depends on the legislative process.

Feasibility of Implementation: High. Many jurisdictions provide property tax credits for a wide range of purposes that are deemed socially beneficial (such as credits for low-income, elderly, disabled, or blind occupants; properties used for charitable or educational purposes; historic preservation; substantial property improvements; and even brownfield clean-up). A credit to promote lead hazard control or other health-related housing improvements would seem to have comparable political appeal.

POTENTIAL OBSTACLES/BARRIERS

Fraudulent use of the credit could occur without proper quality control measures and independent verification of repairs.

ADDITIONAL RESOURCES

N/A

ILLUSTRATION OF STRATEGY IN PRACTICE

Since state-enabling legislation was enacted in 1996, Baltimore has offered a property tax incentive program for owners who complete substantial rehabilitation (greater than 25% of the initial "assessed full market value" of the property) of landmark designated properties and properties located in one of the city's historic districts. The program is not designed, nor has it ever been used, for lead hazard control or other health-related repairs specifically, although such hazards are often corrected incidentally. The assessed tax of the renovated or rehabilitated property remains at the same level as it was before the start of renovation for 10 years. Credit is for 100% of the tax assessment increase due to the improvements made, and is fully transferable to a new owner for the remaining life of the credit—provided the property is certified by CHAP.

Jurisdiction or Target Area: Baltimore, MD

Primary Actor: Baltimore City Commission for Historical and Architectural Preservation (CHAP)

Secondary Actor(s): Maryland State Department of Assessments and Taxation, Baltimore City Department of Finance

Staffing utilized: 1.5 FTE at CHAP run the program. No new staff has been added at the state tax agency or city finance agency, but a tax agency staff person estimates that each agency currently uses as much as 1 FTE staff to do additional data input and record keeping to support this program.

Other resources utilized: N/A

Factors essential to implementation: Implementation requires cooperation among CHAP (accepts, reviews, approves applications and projects), city department of housing and community development (construction permits), state department of taxation (calculates value of tax credit), and city department of finance (issues property tax bills).

Limitations/challenges/problems encountered: Public awareness is limited; the program is publicized mainly through word-of-mouth.

Magnitude of Impact/Potential Impact: Approximately 50,000 properties are eligible. Through the end of 2003, nearly 300 projects have received certification for the tax credit. Some $121.5 million in direct investments have been made in these properties through 2003, and renovations have included structural and major systems repairs, paint removal, and window and trim replacement.

Potential for replication: Moderate.

Contact for Specific Information
Kathleen Kotarba
Executive Director,
Commission for Historical and Architectural Preservation
410-396-4866
kotarba@habc.org

References for additional information
1. www.baltimorecity.gov/government/historic/taxcredit.html
2. www.livebaltimore.com/homebuy/sample.html

SECURE DEDICATED FUNDING FOR CODE ENFORCEMENT

DESCRIPTION OF THE STRATEGY

Code enforcement activities that generate revenues sufficient to cover their costs can avoid the unpredictability of legislative appropriations and minimize the variability in staff or resources that impede enforcement efforts. Governments can adopt ordinances that impose either minimal annual fees or per-unit inspection fees on multi-unit dwellings. Such fees, along with revenues from code enforcement penalties that benefit the program (rather than revert to the jurisdiction's general fund) can provide sufficient resources to expand code inspection programs and improve their effectiveness. States also can make matching grant programs available to local governments to support their building code enforcement efforts.

BENEFITS

Immediate/Direct Results: Reduction in lead hazards in housing resulting from deteriorated paint, and correction of underlying problems, such as roofing or plumbing leaks, that cause paint to flake and peel.
Public Health Benefits: Reduction in the number of children exposed to lead hazards.
Other Indirect/Collateral Benefits: Improvement in the appearance of rental properties and the community in general.

SCOPE OF POTENTIAL IMPACT

Statewide   City- or County-Wide

PRIMARY ACTORS
Building or Code Inspection Agency

KEY PARTNERS
Health Department
Housing Agency
Property Owners

CRITICAL ELEMENTS

Staff requirements: The funding mechanism would not have dedicated staff, but the size of the code enforcement staff will be affected by the amount of dedicated funds it yields.

Other resource requirements: Databases for registering properties and tracking inspections, reinspections, compliance, and penalties.

Institutional capacity required: This strategy requires appropriate legislative or regulatory authority for a code enforcement system and professional trained inspectors. In addition to fines and penalties for non-compliance, an effective code enforcement system should also have a property registration process, regular inspections (every 3-5 years), and re-inspections to ensure compliance.

Cost considerations: If the dedicated funding resource is based on registrations, requirements must be reasonable to allow owners of rental properties to achieve compliance. In addition, the added costs to owners should not be a permissible burden on tenants: the amount that can be passed on to them should be capped.

Timing issues: There are no specific timing issues.

Feasibility of Implementation: Moderate. Feasibility may depend on the willingness and ability of the governmental entity to establish and maintain dedicated funds. In some states and localities, special funds are the norm; in others they are the exception. If the dedicated fund is based on fees and fines, it can be promoted as a payment for services rendered. Some opponents will characterize it as a form of increased taxes on the owners of rental properties.

POTENTIAL OBSTACLES/BARRIERS

One potential obstacle is opposition to new fees if the dedicated fund is established based on fees and fines. Therefore, the fees must be kept to the minimum needed to establish and maintain the fund, and the basis and justification for the new fund must be clear and convincing, based on facts about housing and health conditions.

Second, property owners are likely to object to new or enhanced housing inspections. Public education and outreach must convince decision-makers that (1) inspections are crucial to relieving documented housing conditions that threaten the health and safety of the occupants; and (2) a more professional code enforcement program featuring registration of rental properties, scheduled inspections timed so that property owners can anticipate them, and consistent enforcement processes will provide greater predictability and objectivity as well as accountability for compliance.

Third, the goals of decent housing condition and lead safety must take precedence over zealousness to garner revenues from penalties (to hire more staff to collect more fines, etc.). Orders to comply without financial penalty should be vigorously pursued since in many cases the limited resources of the owner would be better spent on correcting violations rather than paying fines. Fines must be set high enough to motivate property owners to cooperate with enforcement staff as well as preemptively invest in their properties.

ADDITIONAL RESOURCES
N/A

ILLUSTRATION #1 OF STRATEGY IN PRACTICE

The City of Los Angeles has adopted a housing ordinance that requires that every residential rental property with two or more units be inspected on a scheduled basis, currently once every five years. The housing habitability inspection, paid for by a fee of $27.24 per unit per year, covers compliance with codes for fire and life safety, building, electrical, plumbing, heat and ventilation, health, and lead hazards. Lead hazards have been housing code violations since January 2003. Property owners have 30 days to correct violations. Re-inspections are done until the corrective work is done.

Jurisdiction or Target Area: Los Angeles

Primary Actor: Department of Housing

Secondary Actor(s): N/A

Staffing utilized: No information provided.

Other resources utilized: N/A

Factors essential to implementation: The essential components are a professional code enforcement agency, a good database and tracking system, effective outreach and education of property owners and contractors, and consistency of treatment.

Limitations/problems encountered: The program needs to factor in that owners want to/need to recoup investment, and ways to help contractors understand potential liability.

Magnitude of Impact/Potential Impact: Approximately 180,000 units are inspected each year. In a pilot program in one-third of the council districts, inspectors who have been trained in lead safety are citing landlords for visible lead hazards and requiring that all work in pre-1979 buildings that disturbs paint be performed using lead-safe work practices. City inspectors make referrals to the county lead program to document violations. They also refer buildings where children are at-risk to community organizations, which deploy staff to educate tenants to identify and complain of unsafe work practices and to have their children screened.

Potential for replication: Moderate. Cities and counties that have a housing code could adopt a systematic enforcement program using fees or appropriations dedicated to code enforcement. While many codes do not specifically cover deteriorated paint, there are generally other habitability standards that can be cited. Codes inspectors need to be retrained to look at habitability issues, not just building or structural conditions.

Contact for Specific Information
Wayne Durand
Principal Inspector
213-808-8660
wdurand@lahd.lacity.org

References for additional information
1. The City of Los Angeles Housing Department website has an informative summary of the systematic code enforcement program for both tenants and managers/owners. Also, a document called Preparing Residential Property for the Housing Habitability Inspection is helpful for owners and landlords.
www.cityofla.org/lahd/

ILLUSTRATION #2 OF STRATEGY IN PRACTICE

New Jersey requires the registration and inspection every five years of all multiple-unit dwellings. All owners of buildings with three or more units must obtain a Certification of Registration from the Bureau of Housing Inspection. The State then schedules an inspection every fifth year either by BHI inspectors or by local inspectors working under a cooperative agreement with the State. The inspectors issue an inspection report citing violations and the owners have 60 days to correct the violations. Reinspections occur until the problem is corrected; fines may be levied for noncompliance. The inspection includes deteriorated paint on both the interior and exterior. Registration fees and penalties finance the registration/inspection program substantially. The cost of registration is a one-time $10 fee. The inspection fee is a sliding from $16 to $43 per unit, depending on the number of units in the building, every five years.

Jurisdiction or Target Area: State of New Jersey

Primary Actor: Department of Community Affairs, Division of Codes and Standards, Bureau of Housing Inspection (BHI).

Secondary Actor(s): N/A

Staffing utilized: No information provided.

Other resources utilized: N/A

Factors essential to implementation: Registration is the key to success. Once a property is registered, it is possible to contact the owner or the owner's representative. The owner knows the property will be inspected and that it must be maintained. Regular inspections are essential to maintaining properties in a safe condition.

Limitations/problems encountered: It is very difficult to keep up with the constant turnover in ownership of small apartments. The vast majority of properties subject to registration and inspection are three-unit properties. Small property owners are investing for appreciation, not long-term ownership and with little attention to maintenance.

Magnitude of Impact/Potential Impact: 150,000 to 180,000 units are inspected annually.

Potential for replication: Moderate. Other states and localities seeking to replicate New Jersey's approach would need to find a basis for widespread registration that reflect their individual needs and past history. New Jersey laws grew out of a need to regulate tenements in the early 1900s and have gradually evolved since then. Also, the State has a unique relationship with its municipalities that is not common in most states.

Contact for Specific Information

Michael Motich
Supervisory Code Administrator
609-633-6225

References for additional information

1. New Jersey Department of Community Affairs
    www.state.nj.us/dca

LEAD SAFETY AND HEALTHY HOMES STANDARDS

ADOPT STATE AND LOCAL LEAD HAZARD DISCLOSURE LAWS

CERTIFY LEAD SAMPLING TECHNICIANS

ENSURE LEAD SAFETY IN LICENSED CHILD CARE PROGRAMS

ESTABLISH A LEAD-SAFE HOUSING REGISTRY

MAKE LEAD HAZARDS A VIOLATION OF THE HOUSING OR HEALTH CODE

NOTIFY ALL RESIDENTS IN A BUILDING FOUND TO CONTAIN LEAD HAZARDS

PROTECT OCCUPANTS DURING HAZARD REMEDIATION AND RENOVATION WORK

REQUIRE RENTAL PROPERTY OWNERS TO INFORM TENANTS HOW TO REPORT DETERIORATING PAINT

REQUIRE SAFE WORK PRACTICES DURING REMODELING, REPAIR, AND PAINTING

TRAIN PAINTERS, REMODELERS, AND MAINTENANCE STAFF IN LEAD-SAFE WORK PRACTICES

ADOPT STATE AND LOCAL LEAD HAZARD DISCLOSURE LAWS

DESCRIPTION OF THE STRATEGY

Although the federal lead hazard disclosure law requires disclosure of known lead hazards prior to the sale or lease of pre-1978 properties, state and local governments have no authority to enforce it. States and localities seeking to enforce lead hazard disclosure requirements must adopt disclosure laws at the state or local level. Complementing federal law with state or local disclosure requirements can strengthen enforcement and compliance and provide supplemental funding for state and local programs through penalties. Paterson, NJ; Cleveland, OH; Philadelphia, PA; Illinois; Massachusetts; Rhode Island; and Vermont require property owners to disclose lead hazard information to prospective homebuyers and tenants.

State or local laws also can expand the protection afforded by the federal law and can require disclosure of additional information. For example, in multifamily dwellings, the federal law requires disclosure of information only if it pertains to the specific unit being rented or common areas. State and local laws could require that information regarding any unit in the building be disclosed to all prospective tenants. In addition, state and local laws could extend the requirements of the federal law to zero-bedroom dwellings and child care centers.

BENEFITS

Immediate/Direct Results: Homebuyers and tenants receive information about lead-based paint to enable them to make informed housing choices. Since the federal government does not have the staff and resources to cite all violations nationwide, this provides local regulators with an additional "stick" to use with recalcitrant landlords. In addition, states and localities with disclosure laws in place can more easily intervene in federal enforcement cases. (Intervention refers to a party joining in a judicial action already in progress in order to protect an interest or right that may be affected by the proceedings.)

Public Health Benefits: Parents aware that there are or may be lead hazards in their homes are more likely to get their children screened and to take steps to control hazards and reduce their children's exposure to lead. Results of environmental investigations made in response to a poisoned child are required to be disclosed to the next prospective tenant, helping to break the cycle of repeat poisonings. Disclosure requirements will motivate some property owners to address lead hazards.

Other Indirect/Collateral Benefits: States and localities can follow the federal example of pursuing "results-oriented enforcement" of the disclosure law. Federal agencies have entered into settlements with defendants that reduce fines in exchange for agreements from the property owner to invest in lead hazard control in their units and contribute to community-wide prevention efforts. These settlements have resulted in more than $22 million in commitments from landlords to address lead hazards in more than 165,000 units around the country and provided more than $360,000 for community-based projects to combat childhood lead poisoning.

SCOPE OF POTENTIAL IMPACT

Statewide   City- or County-Wide

PRIMARY ACTORS	KEY PARTNERS
Health Department	Housing Agency
Community-based Organizations	Code or Building Inspection Agency
	Local Prosecutors
	Tenants
	Homebuyers

CRITICAL ELEMENTS

Staff requirements: One to two FTEs, possibly over multiple years.

Other resource requirements: While the direct outcome of a disclosure law will be providing families with information they need to make informed housing choices, the reality is that many families living in high-risk housing do not have real housing options. Therefore, the indirect goal of the disclosure requirement is to motivate property owners to go beyond merely providing information about lead hazards and take steps to address them. Resources to assist landlords of low-income properties and owner-occupants, including free trainings in lead-safe work practices and grants and low- or no-interest loans, would help accomplish this goal.

Institutional capacity required: The lead agency, presumably the health or housing department, must have the capacity to enforce the law in order for this strategy to make a meaningful difference. In addition, judges and prosecutors must be educated about lead poisoning and the goals of the law so that settlements and judgments go beyond collecting fines and actually require owners to take measure that will protect tenants.

Cost considerations: This is a low-cost way to motivate owners to invest in lead hazard control. The cost of enforcement can be offset by fees and fines.

Timing issues: The timeline to enact and initially implement a disclosure requirement can be quite long (18 months to 2 years or more), depending on the political climate and the calendar of the city council or state legislature.

Feasibility of Implementation: High, though the successful implementation of this strategy is dependent on legislative approval, which is difficult to predict. Building the support of community-based organizations, tenants, and others concerned about lead poisoning, such as pediatricians, will help achieve passage.

POTENTIAL OBSTACLES/BARRIERS

Landlords, property management companies, and real estate agents may oppose this legislation. In addition, other agencies that need to be involved, such as inspection, code, building, and judicial agencies, may be resistant to taking on what they view as new responsibilities.

ADDITIONAL RESOURCES

1. Contacts for Cases Not Illustrated
   Illinois: Gary Flentge, Illinois Lead and Asbestos Director, 217-782-3517, gflentge@idph.state.il.us.
   Paterson, NJ: Joe Surowiec, Lead Program Coordinator, 973-321-1277, ext. 277.
   Philadelphia: Dick Tobin, 215-685-2788, Richard.tobin@phila.gov
   Vermont: Amy Sayre, VT Health Department, 802-863-7388, asayre@vdh.state.vt.us.

2. Alliance for Healthy Homes, *Model State/Local Lead Disclosure Law*, 2003.
   www.afhh.org/res/res_pubs/disclosure_model_law.pdf
3. Alliance for Healthy Homes, *State and Local Lead Hazard Disclosure Laws*, 2003.
   www.afhh.org/res/res_pubs/disclosure_State%20_Local_Laws.pdf
4. U.S. Department of Housing and Urban Development website
   www.hud.gov/offices/lead/disclosurerule/index.cfm.
5. Illinois Disclosure Law: 410 ILL. COMP. STAT. 45/9.1

6.   Massachusetts Disclosure Law: MASS. GEN. LAWS. ch. 111, § 197A

7.   Rhode Island Disclosure Law: R.I. GEN. LAWS § 23-24.6-16

8.   Paterson, NJ Disclosure Law: PATERSON, N.J. CODE, § 351-3 to -9

9.   Philadelphia, PA Disclosure Law: PHILADELPHIA, PA., HEALTH CODE § 6-803

10. Vermont Disclosure Law: VSA TITLE 18, CH 38, § 176 2

ILLUSTRATION OF STRATEGY IN PRACTICE

In August 2004, the Cleveland City Council passed a new lead-based paint ordinance which, among other important provisions, establishes city lead hazard disclosure requirements and penalties. The ordinance gives the Cleveland Department of Public Health authority to pursue criminal penalties (up to $5,000 per violation) against property owners who fail to distribute the EPA lead hazard information pamphlet, disclose the known presence and location of any lead-based paint or hazard, or fulfill other duties under the federal lead hazard disclosure law.

Jurisdiction or Target Area: Cleveland

Primary Actor: Cleveland Childhood Lead Poisoning Prevention Program (CLPPP)

Secondary Actor: Cleveland Law Department

Staffing utilized: It is estimated that approximately 1 FTE was needed over 12-18 months to conduct background research on other state and local lead laws; draft the legislation; build political support for the new law (including meetings with the Mayor and housing officials); and see it through the legislative process. The director of the CLPPP and a lawyer in the Law Department were the two primary staff who worked on the legislation. The staffing pattern to implement this local disclosure law has not been determined.

Other resources utilized: The program conducted research to review other state and local lead poisoning prevention laws and to survey HUD grantees to learn how they handle properties. The program used the Wisconsin law as a model.

Factors essential to implementation: Political support for the law was essential to its passage. In this case, the Mayor's support of the ordinance assured the support of the Housing Director and Housing Commissioner, both of whom are effective and influential.

Limitations/challenges/problems encountered: The actual implementation and enforcement of the law will depend on having adequate resources and effective communication and coordination between the health and housing departments.

Magnitude of Impact/Potential Impact: There are 178,000 homes in Cleveland built before 1978 that will be affected by the disclosure law. Of those, it is estimated that 120,000 (60%) contain lead hazards and would be candidates for enforcement.

Potential for replication: High.

Contacts for Specific Information

Jonathon Brandt	Shirley Tomasello
Lead Hazard Control Program Manager	Assistant Director of Law
216-664-4939	216-664-3776
jbrandt@city.cleveland.oh.us	stomasello@city.cleveland.oh.us

References for additional information
N/A

CERTIFY LEAD SAMPLING TECHNICIANS

DESCRIPTION OF THE STRATEGY

Testing for lead-contaminated dust is a critical tool for advancing lead poisoning prevention—both to ensure that lead hazards are not left behind after work that disturbs or repairs painted surfaces and to help to identify lead hazards in high-risk properties for corrective action. Home inspectors, community development corporations, public housing authorities, community-based organizations, housing code and HQS inspectors, and public health nurses can use lead dust testing to advance prevention efforts. HUD's lead-safe housing rule accepts clearance by a state-certified lead sampling technician (LST) after non-abatement work. Further, EPA has developed a six-hour training course for LSTs, sponsored its delivery in several communities, and initiated its translation into Spanish. To help make dust testing services by certified personnel more readily available, ten states certify the LST as a free-standing discipline within their EPA-authorized lead programs: Indiana, Iowa, Kentucky, Maine, Michigan, Minnesota, New Hampshire, Ohio, Vermont, and Wisconsin.

BENEFITS

Immediate/Direct Results: By certifying lead sampling technicians as a free-standing discipline, states can greatly enhance local capacity for lead dust testing. Trained LSTs are already qualified to perform initial checks to detect lead hazards in housing. With certification, they can conduct clearance following non-abatement lead hazard reduction activities or renovations under the HUD lead-safe housing rule and by state regulation. Increasing the pool of qualified individuals who can perform lead dust testing can help states to comply with HUD's regulation, which requires clearance following rehab work or lead hazard reduction activities in federally-owned or assisted pre-1978 housing, and can advance state-initiated clearance requirements after non-abatement projects.

Public Health Benefits: Certifying LSTs can significantly increase opportunities for primary prevention. Because LST training requirements are not onerous, and requirements for entry into the discipline are minimal, persons from a wide range of professions can obtain LST certification and incorporate lead dust testing into their work. For example, housing code inspectors can routinely perform dust sampling when a visual inspection in pre-1978 housing reveals potential hazards, and community-based organizations can document lead hazards in high-risk housing and use the data in organizing and advocacy campaigns to seek solutions.

Other Indirect/Collateral Benefits: In 2001, EPA issued standards identifying dangerous levels of lead in paint, dust, and soil. These standards provide uniform benchmarks for stakeholders to use in making informed decisions regarding lead hazards. Certifying LSTs helps to facilitate the widespread use of the standards, since the testing required to determine compliance with the standards will be more accessible and affordable than a risk assessment.

SCOPE OF POTENTIAL IMPACT

Statewide

PRIMARY ACTORS

Health Department

KEY PARTNERS

Housing Agency
Code or Building Inspection Agency
Community-based Organizations
Property Owners
Tenants

CRITICAL ELEMENTS

Staff requirements: States that already have EPA-authorized certification programs in place for lead abatement workers and supervisors, risk assessors, lead inspectors, and project designers will be able to add approval of certifications for LSTs with a nominal amount of staffing.

Other resource requirements: Training materials, testing material samples for practice in lead sampling.

Institutional capacity required: In some states, the laws establishing EPA-authorized certification programs may need to be amended to accommodate LST certification. Elsewhere, agencies administering EPA-authorized programs will only need to promulgate regulations detailing LST certification requirements. Accredited training providers may need to develop LST training programs, but states should be able to approve their plan to use the EPA model course.

Cost considerations: Once a LST certification program is underway, the increased availability of lead dust testing will bring the cost of that service down significantly.

Timing issues: Assuming the statutory authority to certify LSTs is in place, as much as a year may be required to adopt regulations. Individuals typically are certified as LSTs for one or two years and can easily extend their certification through renewal.

Feasibility of Implementation: High. Certifying LSTs as a free-standing discipline is readily achievable in states with EPA-authorized certification programs. In states not currently authorized by EPA to administer certification, sampling technicians who are certified by other states can perform non-abatement clearance in accordance with HUD regulations.

POTENTIAL OBSTACLES/BARRIERS

Confusion or perceived competitive interests may interfere in consideration of certifying LSTs. The benefits of diversifying and expanding capacity need to be communicated.

ADDITIONAL RESOURCES

N/A

ILLUSTRATION OF STRATEGY IN PRACTICE

In 2001, the State of Vermont promulgated regulations that permit the licensing of lead sampling technicians, completing a process that took roughly one year. Candidates are required to attend a five-hour training course designed to give them hands-on experience in conducting visual assessments and taking dust wipe samples, as well as sample submission, lab results interpretation, and other skills. To obtain a license, candidates must pass an exam at the end of the course. Lead sampling technician licenses must be renewed annually. For technicians working for private firms, the license fee is $150 per year; however, public employees and employees of non-profit organizations that are not working commercially can have the fee waived. Licenses or certifications obtained in other states can also be used in Vermont. Lead sampling technicians in Vermont are allowed to perform a well-defined set of duties—they can conduct clearance testing following interim controls, renovations, remodeling, and ongoing maintenance. Sampling technicians cannot perform clearance testing after an abatement project or conduct random dust wipe sampling in multifamily properties.

Jurisdiction or Target Area: Vermont

Primary Actor: Vermont Department of Health

Secondary Actor(s): N/A

Staffing utilized: No new staff was required for the implementation of this strategy. Staff at the Vermont Health Department expended between thirty and forty hours making the needed changes in the Vermont Regulations for Lead Control. Since the adoption of these changes in 2001, no additional staff time has been needed, since the licensing process is integrated into the existing system of licensing asbestos and lead professionals.

Other resources utilized: N/A

Factors essential to implementation: The mandates for clearance testing following lead-safe renovation and remodeling.

Limitations/challenges/problems encountered: None.

Magnitude of Impact/Potential Impact: Since 2001, approximately 50 lead sampling technicians have been licensed in the state of Vermont. Technicians have come from a number of sectors, including local government agencies, community-based organizations, and private industry.

Potential for replication: The potential for replication is high.

Contacts for Specific Information

Vernon Nelson
Vermont Department of Health
802-865-7784
vnelson@vdh.state.vt.us

Ron Rupp
Vermont Housing and Conservation Board
802-828-2912
rrupp@vhcb.state.vt.us

References for additional information
1. Vermont Regs. for Lead Control, Rules 4.3.3.I. and 9.4.
   www.healthyvermonters.info/rules/VRLCFINAL0912.pdf

ENSURE LEAD SAFETY IN LICENSED CHILD CARE PROGRAMS

DESCRIPTION OF THE STRATEGY

Protecting children in child care settings is an essential complement to preventing exposure in the home environment. Requiring property owners of child care programs to certify annually that the program used essential maintenance practices during the previous year will prevent the occurrence of lead hazards. This certification is required for issuance or renewal of the program's child care license and must be filed with the program's insurance carrier.

BENEFITS

Immediate/Direct Results: Once implemented, the program should result in direct and substantial reductions in lead hazards and deteriorated paint at child care programs covered by the regulations.

Public Health Benefits: If a child care facility has lead hazards, children served by the program are likely to become lead poisoned. In addition, since these children may not be considered at high-risk for lead poisoning, they may not be identified under the targeted screening programs used in many states. Reducing lead hazards in child care programs will benefit all of the children who use the program's services.

Other Indirect/Collateral Benefits: The program should raise awareness of lead hazards for the families that use the child care program as the program cleans up problems or proudly declares that it has any potential problems under control.

SCOPE OF POTENTIAL IMPACT

There are 100,000 licensed child care programs nationally serving children under six years old. According to the First National Environmental Health Survey of Child Care Programs, 14 percent of licensed child care programs in the United States have significant lead-based paint hazards – primarily deteriorated lead-based paint. 470,000 children attend these programs. For programs in buildings built before 1960, the rate is 26 percent. For programs where the majority of the children are African American, the rate is 30 percent.

Statewide—State regulation needed.
City- or County-Wide—County or city regulation needed.

PRIMARY ACTORS	KEY PARTNERS
Health Department	Code or Building Inspection Agency
Human and Family Services Agency	Housing Agency
	Property Owners
	Child Care Providers
	Parents

CRITICAL ELEMENTS

Staff requirements: The program will take at least one year to develop, including adoption of laws or rules, development of coalitions, and production of outreach materials. It will take approximately 0.2 FTE to prepare the program, educate child care providers, and manage the program for the first two to three years. In addition, inspectors normally conducting the program inspections will need to be trained to address the issue and integrate compliance monitoring for lead into their workload. The additional inspection burden should be minimal—about 15 minutes per site visit.

Other resource requirements: It may help improve compliance if some inspectors are trained and certified or licensed to conduct a clearance examination. If inspectors will be expected to take dust wipe samples, they will need about $50 per facility for lab analysis of samples.

Institutional capacity required: State child care licensing rules will need revision to require the certification. While not essential, statutory authority such as Vermont's will make it easier. The programs will also need access to contractors and maintenance workers trained in lead-safe work practices to ensure that essential maintenance practices for lead safety are properly done. Some inspection staff may need to be qualified as lead sampling technicians to enhance compliance.

Cost considerations: Child care programs often operate on a tight budget. Many programs lack the resources to remedy lead hazards. Unless resources are provided, programs may be confronted with closure. The programs most at risk for lead hazards are the ones most likely to need the resources.

Timing issues: It will take approximately one year to establish the program and build support for it. Full implementation will usually take two more years. Child care programs are busiest—and therefore unavailable—during August and September when children return to school and enrollment adjusts to the changes.

Feasibility of Implementation: Moderate. The program is feasible to implement in jurisdictions with lead hazard control resources to devote to child card facilities, but it will take the support of agency and political leadership since additional requirements will be imposed on child care programs.

POTENTIAL OBSTACLES/BARRIERS

Management support is essential to overcoming concerns by programs and to manage staff reluctance to expand their inspection role and respond to program concerns.

Communities need to be prepared to identify potential resources to address lead hazards and provide technical assistance to help programs obtain and use those resources.

ADDITIONAL RESOURCES

1. National Resource Center for Health and Safety in Child Care—1-800-598-5437
   http://nrc.uchsc.edu
2. First National Environmental Health Survey of Child Care Centers by the U.S. Department of Housing and Urban Development
   www.hud.gov/offices/lead/techstudies/NatlChildCareSurvey_V1_Lead.pdf

ILLUSTRATION OF STRATEGY IN PRACTICE

In 1996, Vermont adopted a law requiring all licensed child care programs, including those operated as "Family Day Care Homes," to perform annual Essential Maintenance Practices (EMPs). The programs certify that they have completed essential maintenance practices to reduce lead hazards during the previous year. EMPs require use of trained people to: stabilize deteriorated paint, use lead safe work practices, and complete annual specialized cleaning. Child-care program directors must post lead warning notices to program clients. In 2001, the child-care program licensing regulations were changed to require this affidavit in order to receive a license.

Jurisdiction or Target Area: Vermont

Primary Actor: Vermont Department of Health, Childhood Lead Poisoning Prevention Program (CLPPP) and Vermont Social and Rehabilitative Services, Child Care Services Division.

Secondary Actor(s): N/A

Staffing utilized: The program took about 0.2 FTE to design and implement but now operates with minimal effort through the child-care licensing program.

Other resources utilized: Vermont has a comprehensive program to train staff and contractors to use lead-safe work practices.

Factors essential to implementation: Laws or regulation requiring affidavit, as well as resources and training for child care programs to understand and use essential maintenance practices.

Limitations/challenges/problems encountered: Integrating the compliance assurance into the standard licensing program and procedures improved compliance and simplified program management.

Magnitude of Impact/Potential Impact: About 2,200 licensed child care programs must submit an affidavit.

Potential for replication: Very high

Contacts for Specific Information

Amy Sayre
Program Director
802-865-7786
asayre@vdh.state.vt.us

Lea Hatch
Child Care Inspector
802-241-1214
lhatch@srs.state.vt.us

References for additional information
1. Vermont Department of Health CLPPP
   www.healthyvermonters.info/hp/lead/leadchildcare.shtml
2. Vermont Social and Rehabilitative Services Child Care Licensing Requirements
   www.state.vt.us/srs/childcare/licensing/license.htm

ESTABLISH A LEAD-SAFE HOUSING REGISTRY

DESCRIPTION OF THE STRATEGY

Cities, states, and community-based organizations can work to create lead-safe housing registries. These registries allow prospective homeowners or tenants to identify those properties that have been deemed "lead-safe" because a lead hazard evaluation performed by an independent, certified person has found that they comply with federal and state lead laws and regulations. Some of these registries are searchable on the Internet. Pilot projects are also exploring the feasibility of creating a networked, nationwide lead-safe housing registry that would be fully integrated and user-friendly on the web. Other published lists also exist, described in the "Publicize Problem Property Owners" building block.

BENEFITS

Immediate/Direct Results: Establishing a lead-safe housing registry allows prospective tenants and buyers quick, free access to information about properties that are lead-safe.

Public Health Benefits: By directing prospective tenants and homeowners to properties that are lead-safe, a registry can steer families with young children toward healthy housing and away from properties that contain lead hazards. This prevents children from being exposed to home-based lead hazards and reduces lead poisoning risks.

Other Indirect/Collateral Benefits: Property owners who are part of the lead-safe housing registry can market their properties as safe for children and families, attract more tenants and homebuyers, and ultimately obtain higher rents and purchase prices.

SCOPE OF POTENTIAL IMPACT

Statewide   Regional
City- or County-Wide

PRIMARY ACTORS

Health Department
Housing Agency
Community Development Agency
Community-based Organizations

KEY PARTNERS

Property Owners
Homeowners

CRITICAL ELEMENTS

Staff requirements: In most instances, existing staff in a local or state health, housing, or community development department or a community-based organization can create and maintain the lead-safe housing registry. Overall, between 0.25 and 0.5 FTE is needed for this strategy, including ongoing monitoring to ensure that properties listed remain lead-safe if they are not lead-free or fully abated.

Other resource requirements: N/A.

Institutional capacity required: Any agency that receives reports of the lead-safe status of rental properties is positioned to create a registry, although publishing this information in a registry may require specific authorizing legislation.

Cost considerations: Costs to administer this strategy will be moderate; many local lead-safe housing registries have been started as part of a HUD Lead Hazard Control grant. A large portion of costs will be felt at start-up; the costs to maintain the housing registry should be low.

Timing issues: There are no distinct timing issues with this strategy.

Feasibility of Implementation: This strategy should be moderately easy to implement and administer.

POTENTIAL OBSTACLES/BARRIERS

Some resistance from landlords and realtors may occur, in objection to the use of public resources to the benefit of owners of lead-safe properties and to the disadvantage of property owners not on the list (or who will have to undergo costly renovations and repairs to qualify). However, public health concerns should outweigh these arguments.

ADDITIONAL RESOURCES

1. For an example of an interactive online housing registry tool that combines information on lead-safe housing with data on housing containing known lead hazards, visit
www.LeadSafeHomes.info

ILLUSTRATION #1 OF STRATEGY IN PRACTICE

Since 1995, Montgomery County, Ohio, has received grant funds from HUD's Office of Healthy Homes and Lead Hazard Control totaling $4.9 million. Like many grantees, Montgomery County targets specific neighborhoods with lead hazard control activities. As part of its overall grant program, the County has established a lead-safe housing registry. Currently, the registry covers the City of Dayton, the City of Kettering, and several properties scattered throughout Montgomery County. The registry distinguishes between owner-occupied and tenant-occupied properties. The county has made the registry available online, complete with photos of selected properties.

Jurisdiction or Target Area: Montgomery County, OH

Primary Actor: Montgomery County Community Development Office

Secondary Actors: Montgomery County Printing Office; City of Kettering; City of Dayton

Staffing utilized: Less than forty hours of staff time was used to establish the registry. Montgomery County's Printing Office, which maintains the county's website, helped post the registry online. Annual updates of the registry take two to four hours of staff time between the Community Development Office and the Printing Office.

Other resources utilized: HUD Lead Hazard Control funds were used for registry start-up.

Factors essential to implementation: Factors essential to implementation of the lead-safe housing registry in Montgomery County included the availability of HUD grant funds and the cooperation of the cities of Kettering and Dayton, as well as assistance from a variety of other parties, including the Sunrise Center, the CityWide Development Corporation, and the Center for Healthy Communities.

Limitations/challenges/problems encountered: There were no significant limitations or challenges encountered in establishing the Montgomery County Lead-Safe Housing Registry.

Magnitude of Impact/Potential Impact: The Montgomery County registry currently lists 102 owner-occupied housing units and 56 rental units as lead-safe.

Potential for replication: Cities and counties that receive state or federal grant funds can easily establish a lead-safe housing registry as part of their overall programs. Eleven counties in California and the City of Long Beach have established similar registries.

Contact for Specific Information

Montgomery County Community Development Office
937-225-6318

References for additional information
1. Montgomery County Lead Hazard Control Program and Lead-Safe Housing Registry
   www.co.montgomery.oh.us/Departments/com&econ/lead.html
2. California's LEAD Safe Rental Registry
   www.csd.ca.gov/leadregistry.html
3. City of Long Beach Lead-Safe Housing Directory
   http://cms.longbeach.gov/health/lead_safe_registry.html

ILLUSTRATION #2 OF STRATEGY IN PRACTICE

The Lead Safe Housing Registry in Maryland is a product of the Coalition to End Childhood Lead Poisoning, a nonprofit organization headquartered in Baltimore. The registry is a statewide list of currently available rental properties that, according to the records of the Maryland Department of the Environment, are in compliance with state and federal lead safety standards. Properties on the registry are designated as having undergone a full risk reduction or as being lead-safe or lead-free. The list is unique in that it shows only properties currently available for rent, along with the type of unit (apartment, townhouse, etc.), some of the amenities, the amount of the security deposit, the total rent per month, and whether the unit is eligible for subsidy under HUD's Section 8 Housing Choice Voucher program. In addition, some of the properties listed on the housing registry are considered affordable housing.

Jurisdiction or Target Area: Maryland

Primary Actor: Coalition to End Childhood Lead Poisoning

Secondary Actors: N/A

Staffing utilized: The Coalition did a lot of preliminary groundwork in establishing Maryland's lead-safe housing registry. 1-2 FTE were temporarily needed for this process. Maintaining and updating the list on a biweekly basis requires 0.25 FTE.

Other resources utilized: N/A

Factors essential to implementation: The initial and ongoing cooperation of the state of Maryland has been essential to the Coalition in implementing this strategy.

Limitations/challenges/problems encountered: The Coalition has encountered several challenges in making its registry as complete as possible. The State of Maryland is prohibited by law from making public an inventory of properties owned by a specific landlord or leasing company for any purpose, so the Coalition must list units on an individual basis. Also, although the Coalition attempts to provide a large selection of lead-safe affordable housing, these properties are in short supply. Developing the housing registry for the less urban sections of Maryland (i.e. outside the Baltimore metro area and the Washington, DC suburbs) is another challenge for the Coalition.

Magnitude of Impact/Potential Impact: The impact of this registry is statewide. Properties from every county can be included on the registry. Because the registry can include a limitless number of affordable housing units, it can have positive impacts on low-income families in Maryland.

Potential for replication: In states where statutes or regulations allow or require lead-safe housing certification, a community-based or statewide nonprofit organization with sufficient resources could easily replicate this housing registry, though it may be more challenging to establish statewide registries in more rural states than in those with large metro areas.

Contact for Specific Information
G. Wesley Stewart
Coalition to End Childhood Lead Poisoning
410-534-6447, ext. 13
gwstewart@leadsafe.org

References for additional information
1.   Maryland's Statewide Lead-Safe Housing Registry
     www.leadsafe.org/Coalition_services/Housing/Housing_index.html

ILLUSTRATION #3 OF STRATEGY IN PRACTICE

The Wisconsin Lead-Free/Lead-Safe Registry is a listing of houses, apartments, day care facilities, and other buildings that meet the state's lead-free or lead-safe property standard. The lead-free standard is met when a property does not contain lead-based paint. A lead-safe property is one that does not contain lead hazards, such as peeling, chipping, or flaking lead-based paint.

A property owner may apply to be added to the registry by obtaining a lead-free or lead-safe certificate, which is issued following an inspection by a certified lead inspector or risk assessor. Lead-safe certificates are valid for a set period of time as determined by DHFS; lead-free certificates do not expire.

The Lead-Free/Lead-Safe Registry is posted online; the .pdf file is updated whenever a significant number of properties have been added. The registry is organized by county and lists the address of the property, whether the property is lead-free or lead-safe, and contact information for the property owner or the owner's representative. DHFS is working to make the information available in an interactive format through the Wisconsin Asbestos Lead Database Online (WALDO). While no definite timeline has been set, ultimately the database will be located at http://dhfs.wisconsin.gov/waldo/.

Jurisdiction or Target Area: Wisconsin

Primary Actor: Wisconsin Department of Health and Family Services (DHFS)

Secondary Actors: N/A

Staffing utilized: 1 FTE

Other resources utilized: N/A

Factors essential to implementation: The policy requiring DFHS access to addresses of lead-safe/lead-free properties and the availability of these addresses to the public has been crucial to the success and timeliness of the registry.

Limitations/challenges/problems encountered: Publishing the WALDO database online has been the main challenge for DHFS. While an online version currently exists to collect input from property owners, it is complicated and too cumbersome for display and interactive activity by website visitors. DHFS is currently seeking funding to make the database more user-friendly and fully available to the public.

Magnitude of Impact/Potential Impact: The impact of this registry is statewide.

Potential for replication: Very high in states where statutes or regulations require lead-safe and/or lead-free housing certification.

Contacts for Specific Information

Gail Boushon
Program Coordinator
Wisconsin Dept. of Health and Family Services
Asbestos and Lead Unit
608-261-6876
boushga@dhfs.state.wi.us

Pam Campbell
Regulatory Specialist
Wisconsin Dept. of Health and Family Services
Asbestos and Lead Unit
608-261-6876
campbpj@dhfs.state.wi.us

References for additional information

1. Wisconsin's Statewide Lead-Safe/Lead-Free Housing Registry
   http://dhfs.wisconsin.gov/waldo/Registry/index.htm
2. Wisconsin Rule on Registry of Property with Certificates of Lead–Free Status or Lead–Safe Status, Wis. Admin. Code §§HFS 163.40-163.43
   www.legis.state.wi.us/rsb/code/hfs/hfs163.pdf

MAKE LEAD HAZARDS A VIOLATION
OF THE HOUSING OR HEALTH CODE

DESCRIPTION OF THE STRATEGY

In order to provide the clearest legal basis for code officials to confront lead hazards, local and state codes should state explicitly that deteriorated lead-based paint and dangerous levels of lead in dust and bare soil constitute violations of the housing or health code. Specifically referencing lead hazards in the housing or health code will alert enforcement officials and property owners alike that such hazards constitute code violations and must be corrected. The code can explicitly incorporate EPA's national standard for dangerous levels of lead in paint, dust, and soil that state and local jurisdictions can reference.

BENEFITS

Immediate/Direct Results: Enforcement officials have the authority to mandate repair or abatement and cite property owners who fail to comply.

Public Health Benefits: Children are protected from exposure because hazards are addressed on a pre-emptive basis.

Other Indirect/Collateral Benefits: With the prospect of enforcement and fines, some property owners may be motivated to repair their property before problems occur.

SCOPE OF POTENTIAL IMPACT

Statewide   City- or County-wide

PRIMARY ACTORS	KEY PARTNERS
Inspection, Code, or Building Agency	State or local legislators

CRITICAL ELEMENTS

Staff requirements: Since adding lead hazards supplements existing code enforcement programs' authority, no additional staffing would be needed.

Other resource requirements: N/A

Institutional capacity required: The initial requirement is local or state legislation that names deteriorated lead-based paint and dangerous levels of lead in dust and bare soil as code violations. Implementation requires training for code staff in the identification of lead hazards and certification to become lead sampling technicians, lead-based paint inspectors, or risk assessors.

Cost considerations: None identified.

Time issues: None

Feasibility of Implementation: High. Adding lead hazards to the housing code is not difficult to implement.

POTENTIAL OBSTACLES/BARRIERS

The strategy has limited usefulness if local jurisdictions do not have the budget or staff to investigate and enforce violations.

ADDITIONAL RESOURCES

1. EPA Section 403, 15 U.S.C. 2683 (40 CFR 745)

ILLUSTRATION OF STRATEGY IN PRACTICE

The Town of Manchester's Property Maintenance Code requires that interior and exterior lead-based paint must either be maintained in a condition free from peeling, chipping, and flaking or be removed or covered in an appropriate manner. Cases involving lead-based paint violations are referred to the health and building departments to pursue compliance with state and federal regulations. If a child under six years of age resides in a property with deteriorated, flaking, or loose paint conditions, dust wipe samples are collected. If lab analysis results reveal lead hazards, repairs are ordered and the property owner is referred to the Lead Abatement Project, which may provide financial support to complete the repairs. Participants in the program are required to obtain lead safe work practices training.

Jurisdiction or Target Area: Manchester, CT

Primary Actor: Department of Health, Lead Abatement Project, in conjunction with the city's Code Enforcement Unit.

Secondary Actor(s): N/A

Staffing utilized: Only 0.2 FTE is available to address Property Maintenance Code complaints. One full time Property Maintenance Inspector, with support staff, would be needed to proactively address lead hazards in a town the size of Manchester.

Other resources utilized: N/A

Factors essential to implementation: Strong partnership with a childhood lead poisoning prevention program and enough staff to implement property maintenance code.

Limitations/challenges/problems encountered: Generally, Code Department personnel focus primarily on new construction and only react to property maintenance complaints, so there is a need for on-going education and advocacy about lead hazards in older properties. Nonetheless, a partnership between the building inspectors and the Lead Abatement Project has made a difference.

Magnitude of Impact/Potential Impact: By making lead hazards part of the Property Maintenance Code, Manchester has institutionalized the importance of recognizing and addressing them. This is an essential step in eradicating lead poisoning, particularly in an area where 93 percent of the housing is at risk for lead hazards.

Potential for replication: High. The housing code provision is not difficult to implement, but to reach its full potential impact, the jurisdiction should have sufficient resources for code inspection and enforcement.

Contacts for Specific Information

Sue Heller
Administrator, Lead Abatement Project
860-647-3288
sue41@ci.manchester.ct.us

John Hogan
Chief Building Inspector
860-647-3052
John21@ci.manchester.ct.us

References for additional information

1. Town of Manchester, Code of Ordinances, Property Maintenance Code §7-305.4 et seq.

NOTIFY ALL RESIDENTS IN A BUILDING FOUND TO CONTAIN LEAD HAZARDS

DESCRIPTION OF THE STRATEGY

The presence of lead hazards in one unit of a multi-family building is a strong indication that other units in the building also contain hazards. Through statutes or code, hazard assessment staff can be given the authority to notify, or rental property owners can be required to notify, all building residents of any evaluation, inspection, other hazard determination, hazard reduction activities, or clearance testing performed in the building. By putting all occupants on notice when hazards are identified, residents can take steps to protect their children from lead poisoning.

BENEFITS

Immediate/Direct Results: Occupants will become aware of existing lead hazards and may be motivated to seek an assessment or corrective action in their own unit. As a result, other hazards in the same building will be identified and remediated before more children are poisoned.

Public Health Benefits: Expand awareness and education of lead hazards among residents.

Other Indirect/Collateral Benefits: Notification of all tenants provides an opportunity for community building among residents.

SCOPE OF POTENTIAL IMPACT

Statewide   City- or County-Wide

PRIMARY ACTORS

Code or Housing Inspection Agency

KEY PARTNERS

Tenants

CRITICAL ELEMENTS

Staff requirements: Approximately 0.05 FTE.

Other resource requirements: N/A

Institutional capacity required: Hazard assessment personnel must have the authority to notify all residents when a unit located in the same structure is cited for lead hazards.

Cost considerations: None listed

Timing issues: None

Feasibility of Implementation: Very high. This is a simple, low-cost education and outreach tool.

POTENTIAL OBSTACLES/BARRIERS

Non-English-speaking tenants need notice and educational materials in the appropriate language.

ADDITIONAL RESOURCES

N/A

ILLUSTRATION OF STRATEGY IN PRACTICE

San Francisco's Health Code gives the Department of Public Health the authority to notify all residents of a building where an investigation documents lead hazards in any unit in that building. When an inspection reveals lead hazards, the environmental health inspector gives the property owner a report highlighting the hazard and where it is located and instructs the property owner to copy and distribute the notice to all tenants in the building. In order to ensure all tenants actually receive the notice, the department also distributes copies, along with lead hazard educational materials. The materials are available in Chinese, Spanish, and English.

Jurisdiction or Target Area: San Francisco

Primary Actor: San Francisco Department of Public Health, Children's Environmental Health Promotion Program.

Secondary Actor(s): N/A

Staffing utilized: 0.05 FTE to prepare the photocopies, assemble the literature, and distribute it to tenants.

Other resources utilized: A photocopier and educational literature.

Factors essential to implementation: The Health Code gives inspectors the authority to notify all tenants.

Limitations/challenges/problems encountered: The challenge involves distributing the flyers and ensuring that materials are provided in the appropriate language for the tenants.

Magnitude of Impact/Potential Impact: The Children's Environmental Health Promotion Program has not yet collected data on this strategy's impact, but inspectors consider it a strategy complementary to their overall environmental health promotion. Distributing notice to all tenants is another way to build awareness and reinforces the seriousness of San Francisco's lead problem.

Potential for replication: Very high. This strategy is easily replicated with very little cost incurred.

Contact for Specific Information
Karen Yu
Senior Environmental Health Inspector
415-252-3957
karen.yu@sfdph.org

References for additional information
1. San Francisco Health Code Art. 26, §1626(e)
2. San Francisco Building Code §3606.4

PROTECT OCCUPANTS
DURING HAZARD REMEDIATION AND RENOVATION WORK

DESCRIPTION OF THE STRATEGY

Generally, occupants of homes that contain lead-based paint should be temporarily relocated to lead-safe housing before the start of lead hazard control work, or renovation or remodeling work that disturbs more than a small area of lead-based paint, and they should not return until the work is completed and the work site has been vacuum cleaned and wet washed and passed clearance.

Relocation is not necessary if work area containment is practiced and either only a few square feet of paint will be disturbed or the work can be completed in a few days while occupants stay out of the work area.

Temporary relocation can be carried out most efficiently and costs minimized by (a) ensuring that paint-disturbing work is completed as quickly as possible; (b) occupants are fully advised in writing of the necessity of not returning until the dwelling has been thoroughly cleaned; and (c) arrangements are made in advance for the protection and security of occupants' belongings and for the transportation needs of schoolchildren.

BENEFITS

Immediate/Direct Results: Temporary relocation protects occupants from exposure to lead during such activities.

Public Health Benefits: In areas such as New England, 20% or more of elevated blood lead level cases can be traced to unsafe remodeling or renovation of the child's home. Therefore, ensuring needed relocation could materially reduce childhood lead poisoning.

Other Indirect/Collateral Benefits: Rental property owners and contractors would avoid liability for poisoning children by providing temporary relocation.

SCOPE OF POTENTIAL IMPACT

Statewide   City- or County-Wide

PRIMARY ACTORS

Health Department
Community-based Organizations

KEY PARTNERS

Property Owners
Remodeling and Renovation Contractors

CRITICAL ELEMENTS

Staff requirements: Health and Housing Department staff, supported by community and advocacy organizations, would have to devote time to educating landlords and contractors on the importance of temporary relocation. Contractor training programs should include temporary relocation in training materials. Building permit agencies could review plans for occupied property renovations.

Other resource requirements: Training materials and a database of housing by year built would be required.

Institutional capacity required: Knowledge of the local housing base.

Cost considerations: The cost of temporary relocation should be borne by owners of rental properties. At minimum, state or local agencies could encourage rental property owners to pay for incidental costs, such as transportation and security of occupants' belongings, if occupants arrange to stay with friends or relatives. Some public and private agencies have secured lead-safe apartments and required rental property owners to pay for incidental costs. Where private sector accommodations must be used, relocation costs can be minimized if the agency can establish a public-private partnership with hotels or motels to set aside low-cost rooms for temporary relocation.

In addition, it is conceivable that a temporary relocation requirement will result in rental property owners passing the cost to tenants in the form of higher rent.

Timing issues: N/A

Feasibility of Implementation: High. Encouraging temporary relocation to homes of the occupant's friends or relatives may be one practical way of minimizing costs and ensuring successful implementation. Otherwise, feasibility will depend upon the availability of funds to implement a program.

POTENTIAL OBSTACLES/BARRIERS

It may be very difficult to impose temporary relocation requirements on landlords without the availability of some type of cost-sharing.

ADDITIONAL RESOURCES

N/A

ILLUSTRATION OF STRATEGY IN PRACTICE

This strategy is HUD's temporary relocation policy for federally assisted housing rehabilitation and renovation work. The policy provides for temporary relocation of residents to lead-safe housing during the work period, but it does not require relocation if certain requirements are met. If only a small area of paint will be disturbed; if the work can be completed in one 8-hour work day or within five calendar days, occupants are kept out of the work area, warning signs are placed in each room where work is occurring, and the area is thoroughly cleaned are work is completed; or only outside work is involved, the property owner does not have to relocate the unit's occupants.

Jurisdiction or Target Area: Nationwide federally-assisted housing

Primary Actor: U.S. Dept. of Housing and Urban Development (HUD)

Secondary Actor(s): N/A

Staffing utilized: Staff at more than 1,000 local housing agencies across the U.S. monitor relocation within the context of their more comprehensive grant monitoring.

Other resources utilized: Some agencies allow temporary relocation costs as an eligible expense for housing rehab programs.

Factors essential to implementation: Coordination and cooperation among occupants, property owners, and contractors involved in the rehabilitation and renovation work. It also requires ongoing inspection and enforcement by HUD and local housing agencies.

Limitations/challenges/problems encountered: HUD exempted elderly homeowners from relocation requirements since local agencies reported that this population did not want to be relocated and was considered at low risk.

Magnitude of Impact/Potential Impact: Unknown.

Potential for replication: Moderate

Contact for Specific Information

HUD's Office of Healthy Homes and Lead Hazard Control
202-755-1755

References for additional information

1. HUD Interpretive Guidance on Occupant Relocation
   www.centerforhealthyhousing.org/1012/html/relocation.html
2. HUD regulations on occupant protection
   www.centerforhealthyhousing.org/1012/html/occupant_protection.html

REQUIRE RENTAL PROPERTY OWNERS TO INFORM TENANTS HOW TO REPORT DETERIORATING PAINT

DESCRIPTION OF THE STRATEGY

Requiring property owners to provide information on lead hazards to tenants and to inform tenants how to report deteriorating paint can increase tenant awareness of the risk of lead hazards and assist them if paint deterioration problems develop. Notices can be delivered or mailed to tenants or posted in the building to inform occupants of basic lead hazard control measures, ask them to report deteriorated paint, and provide them with the information necessary to report conditions of concern. This strategy is effective only to the extent that property owners promptly and safely repair deteriorated paint and its causes. This type of notice to tenants is required in Vermont, Rhode Island, and housing subject to HUD's lead-safe housing rule: public housing, housing subsidized by a variety of HUD assistance programs (including the Section 8 Housing Choice Voucher program), and properties that HUD is selling.

BENEFITS

Immediate/Direct Results: This strategy can increase tenant awareness of the risk of lead hazards and increase the likelihood that property owners are made aware if paint deterioration develops, which, in turn, increases the likelihood of corrective action.

Public Health Benefits: Lead exposure is reduced if deteriorated paint is repaired more promptly and in a lead-safe manner.

Other Indirect/Collateral Benefits: Property owners and occupants will become more aware of the hazards associated with deteriorated lead paint and will pay more attention to paint condition. Code enforcement personnel may also pay more attention to deteriorated paint.

SCOPE OF POTENTIAL IMPACT

City- or County-Wide

Specific (Targeted) Population—Notice requirement could be restricted to a higher-risk set of properties, such as pre-1950 rental housing

PRIMARY ACTORS

Health Department

KEY PARTNERS

Code or Building Inspection Agency
Housing Agency
Local Prosecutors
Community-based Organizations
Property Owners
Tenants
Community Members

CRITICAL ELEMENTS

Staff requirements: The requirement to notify could be considered self-enforcing, but governmental enforcement efforts can greatly improve awareness and compliance. Very minimal staffing within a health or code enforcement agency (0.2-0.5 FTE) could create a basic education and outreach program to increase landlord awareness of the requirement. High-profile enforcement actions against egregious violations and/or spot-checking properties for compliance would be a reasonable starting point for additional enforcement efforts. Staffing levels for enforcement could be further increased to the point where additional staff produces diminishing returns. To the extent that increased reporting to landlords of deteriorated paint does not prompt safe repairs by landlords, additional hazard inspection and enforcement may be needed.

Other resource requirements: Additional staff dedicated to ensuring landlord compliance probably could be funded mostly or entirely from penalties assessed against non-complying landlords.

Institutional capacity required: State or local legislation would need to be enacted to create the notice requirement and enforcement authority to ensure compliance.

Cost considerations: This requirement seems cost-effective no matter how passively or aggressively it is enforced. Without enforcement, some compliance will occur at virtually no cost. Additional resources spent on landlord outreach and education and/or enforcement should increase compliance substantially. Penalties against non-compliant landlords would increase in proportion to resources spent on enforcement and cover or at least offset costs of enforcement.

Timing issues: No seasonal or cyclical considerations. Timeline to implement depends on the legislative process.

Feasibility of Implementation: Moderate. The existence of this policy in two states and throughout most federally assisted housing demonstrates its feasibility.

POTENTIAL OBSTACLES/BARRIERS

The impact of this policy is directly related to the degree to which it is promoted and enforced among landlords. Some resources would have to be committed initially in order to demonstrate cost effectiveness of promotion and enforcement. This is most likely to happen if policy makers are shown or convinced that enforcement efforts can pay for themselves.

ADDITIONAL RESOURCES

N/A

ILLUSTRATION OF STRATEGY IN PRACTICE

In 1996, the Vermont Legislature enacted the Essential Maintenance Practices law, which includes a requirement that owners of pre-1978 rental housing and child care facilities "post, in a prominent place … a notice to occupants emphasizing the importance of promptly reporting deteriorated paint to the owner or to the owner's agent. The notice shall include the name, address, and telephone number of the owner or the owner's agent." The law also requires owners of pre-1978 rental housing to annually submit an Affidavit of Performance attesting to compliance with this and the other requirements to the Vermont Department of Health.

Jurisdiction or Target Area: Vermont

Primary Actor: Vermont Housing and Conservation Board

Secondary Actor(s): Vermont Department of Health

Staffing utilized: There is no dedicated funding or staff for this strategy. Presently the entire law is being implemented within the Vermont Department of Health's (VDH) existing budget, utilizing less than 1 FTE. It is estimated that 2 FTEs are needed to track and respond to complaints and apparent non-compliance.

Other resources utilized: Required training course, fact sheets, associated forms, guidance, and affidavit filing system.

Factors essential to implementation: Coordination between Vermont Department of Health and Vermont Housing and Conservation Board is essential, as is sufficient staffing to ensure compliance.

REQUIRE RENTAL PROPERTY OWNERS TO INFORM TENANTS HOW TO REPORT DETERIORATING PAINT

Limitations/challenges/problems encountered: Although VDH is charged with implementing the law and keeping records, no money is appropriated for these activities or for enforcement. VDH does not have the resources to conduct quality control on affidavits to verify they are correctly completed or to physically check dwellings to confirm compliance. Currently, VDH attempts to resolve complaints informally but does not use its statutory power to penalize non-compliant landlords. VDH has never issued a health order to address violations of the law—even after the infraction caused a child to be lead poisoned. Failure to prosecute even the most egregious cases means there are essentially no negative consequences to ignoring the law.

Magnitude of Impact/Potential Impact: Approximately 30-40 percent of Vermont's pre-1978 rental housing units have affidavits on file at VDH that claim compliance. According to officials, the lack of any comprehensive listing of rental properties hinders the agency's ability to get a precise picture of compliance. However, Vermont is poised to have a larger impact in the future, and other jurisdictions with more staff availability could be even more effective.

Potential for replication: Moderate

Contact for Specific Information
Ron Rupp
Director, Lead-Based Paint Hazard Reduction Program
Vermont Housing and Conservation Board
802-828-2912
rrupp@vhcb.state.vt.us

References for additional information
1. The Vermont Lead Law (Vermont Statutes, Title 18, Chapter 38)
   www.leg.state.vt.us/statutes/sections.cfm?Title=18&Chapter=038
2. Vermont Housing and Conservation Board's "Lead-Safe Vermont" web site
   www.leadsafevermont.org
3. Vermont Tenants, Inc. "Lead Safety" web page
   www.cvoeo.org/vti/leadInfo_introduction.htm

REQUIRE SAFE WORK PRACTICES
DURING REMODELING, REPAIR, AND PAINTING

DESCRIPTION OF THE STRATEGY

Banning unsafe work practices and requiring basic safeguards for remodeling and paint repair work are key to preventing childhood lead poisoning in older housing. Banning unsafe methods of removing paint will sharply reduce the amount of lead contaminated dust that would otherwise be generated. The unsafe methods that should be prohibited include: dry sanding or scraping; open flame burning; operating a heat gun above 1100 degrees; machine sanding without a HEPA attachment; and stripping in poorly ventilated areas using volatile strippers on surfaces containing lead-based paint. Requiring precautions such as work area containment and careful post-work cleaning will prevent the dispersal of any lead-contaminated dust that might be generated. When coupled with occupant protection activities, adherence to lead-safe work practices for routine remodeling and repair work can help prevent children's exposure to lead dust hazards.

BENEFITS

Immediate/Direct Results: Homes that are being remodeled, repaired, or repainted are less likely to pose lead dust hazards if contractors refrain from unsafe work methods that generate lead dust and follow basic precautions while performing work that disturbs paint in older homes.

Public Health Benefits: Following lead-safe work practices will materially reduce risks to children living in older homes that are undergoing repairs or renovation. In many areas, such as New England, up to 20% of lead poisoning cases can be attributed to unsafe remodeling or renovation activities.

Other Indirect/Collateral Benefits: A requirement for using lead-safe work practices would also reduce exposure of workers, and potentially their children, to dangerous levels of lead dust.

SCOPE OF POTENTIAL IMPACT

A requirement for using lead-safe work practices could be implemented statewide or at the county or city level. Similar requirements already apply to all remodeling, rehab, and paint repair projects in HUD-assisted housing and properties rehabilitated using HUD funds.

PRIMARY ACTORS	KEY PARTNERS
Health Department	
Housing/Community Development Agency	
Remodeling and Renovation Contractors	
Community-based Organizations	

CRITICAL ELEMENTS

Staff Requirements: Health and Housing Department staff, supported by community and advocacy organizations, would have to devote time to inform legislative efforts to enact lead-safe work practices requirements.

Other resource requirements: N/A

Institutional Capacity Required: To foster contractor and worker capacity and increase compliance, public agencies should offer free or low-cost training in lead-safe work practices, adapting state-of-the-art curriculum (notably the 5.5 hour training course developed by HUD and EPA in 2003) to cover any additional state or local requirements. Training facilities, such as community colleges and vocational technical programs, should also be encouraged to offer training in lead-safe work practices.

Cost Considerations: Because some banned work practices, such as machine sanding, reduce labor time in surface preparation, painting contractors and their clients would bear marginal increased costs.

Timing Issues: Developing and implementing systems to train remodeling contractors, painters, and maintenance workers will take time.

Feasibility of Implementation: Moderate. Training to build lead safety capacity can start before requirements are in place. Health department leadership will accelerate acceptance and enactment of lead-safe work practices requirements. Substantial support from community and advocacy organizations will help. Property owner and contractor associations should be asked to participate in developing the statute, ordinance, or code amendment to offset their likely opposition. Compliance will grow over time, because most contractors are law-abiding or interested in avoiding legal liability and are responsive to consumer awareness and demand for lead safety. Success is more likely in areas with a relatively high incidence of lead poisoning and broad public awareness.

POTENTIAL OBSTACLES/BARRIERS

The main obstacles are likely to be the opposition of property owners and contractors to enactment of requirements for lead-safe work practices.

ADDITIONAL RESOURCES
N/A

ILLUSTRATION OF STRATEGY IN PRACTICE

In 2001, the City of New Orleans enacted an ordinance that prohibits unsafe work practices during work on metal structures and buildings built before 1978. It requires that contaminated debris be contained within barriers and that visible paint chips be cleaned after completion of work. It also requires that tenants, neighbors, workers, and government agencies be notified that work on interior and exterior painted surfaces will take place and forbids retaliatory evictions. Enforcement is mostly by complaint and is more effective for work on exteriors that are evident to neighbors. The city is authorized to issue notices of violation, to require remediation of any lead-based paint hazards generated by unsafe work, and to require a risk assessment before resumption of work.

Jurisdiction or Target Area: New Orleans

Primary Actor: Health Department and Department of Safety and Permits

Secondary Actor(s): N/A

Staffing utilized: 0.25 FTE

Other resources utilized: N/A

Factors Essential to Implementation: A coalition of physicians and community advocates worked with the city's administration to develop the ordinance, which was passed in the wake of a survey finding that 25 percent of children screened at city-operated clinics had elevated blood lead levels. City departments and advocates must ensure wide publicity and education so that tenants and neighbors will report violations and so that violations will be vigorously pursued.

Limitations/challenges/problems encountered: The ordinance only applies to lead-based paint, which allows painters and owners to submit an unleaded paint chip to circumvent all requirements.

Magnitude of Impact/Potential Impact: The introduction of notices of work on older buildings has alerted residents to the dangers of unsafe renovation and remodeling. Contractors are being more careful when doing exterior work.

Potential for replication: High

Contact for Specific Information
Jerry McRaney
Assistant Chief Building Inspector, Department of Safety and Permits
504-565-6130

References for additional information
N/A

TRAIN PAINTERS, REMODELERS, AND MAINTENANCE STAFF IN LEAD-SAFE WORK PRACTICES

DESCRIPTION OF THE STRATEGY

Research makes clear that routine work disturbing painted surfaces can create lead dust hazards. "Basic training" in lead-safe work practices is now readily available to reach painters, remodelers, and maintenance staff to educate them on the work practices that are needed to control, contain, and clean up any lead dust generated by their work. A new HUD/EPA 5½-hour "basic training" course includes valuable "hands-on" exercises and can be easily taught in most localities.

BENEFITS

Immediate/Direct Results: Attendees will have the knowledge and skills necessary to use lead-safe work practices immediately. These practices will reduce lead hazards during renovation and maintenance work.

Public Health Benefits: As the lead-safe work practices learned by attendees are used on maintenance and renovation projects, fewer children will be exposed to lead-based paint hazards in their homes.

Other Indirect/Collateral Benefits: Lead-safe work practices will become far more widespread as more professionals are trained to teach the class. This will help to avoid the creation of lead-based paint hazards and will help reduce hazards that already exist. Lead-safe work practices require, among other things, extensive dust control during work and thorough cleaning once a job is completed. This can significantly reduce dust levels and other respiratory irritants in remodeled homes and apartments.

SCOPE OF POTENTIAL IMPACT

Statewide	Regional (e.g. multi-county)
City- or County-Wide	Neighborhood/Community
Specific (Targeted) Populations—Contractors	

PRIMARY ACTORS

Code or Building Inspection Agency
Housing Agency

KEY PARTNERS

Property Owners
Contractors
Painters
Maintenance Workers
Homeowners

CRITICAL ELEMENTS

Staff requirements: This strategy will require staff time to conduct trainings and follow-up with attendees. A good trainer will need two days to become familiar with the curriculum.

Other resource requirements: Lead-safe work practices materials will need to be copied for each attendee. In addition, hands-on supplies will be needed.

Institutional capacity required: An experienced trainer is needed to teach the class. Statutes, regulations, and/or municipal codes should ideally include standards for training requirements for painters and remodelers.

Cost considerations: Cost will mostly involve staff time and training materials. These expenses should be low or moderate.

Timing issues: This strategy would require some short-duration outreach.

Feasibility of Implementation: Very high. Implementation of this strategy should be feasible in almost all jurisdictions.

POTENTIAL OBSTACLES/BARRIERS

There should be few, if any, obstacles to impede implementation of this strategy.

ADDITIONAL RESOURCES

N/A

ILLUSTRATION OF STRATEGY IN PRACTICE

In 1991, the State of Rhode Island passed a comprehensive lead law designed to protect children from lead poisoning. Included as part of that law is a strategy that requires all painters, remodelers, and others who are working with lead-based paint, or who seek to control existing lead hazards, to obtain training in lead-safe work practices.

The Department refers all applicants for certification on lead-safe work practices to a list of training providers. It also provides the general public with resource information on lead-safe work practices. This information is available through the Department's Family Health Information Line.

Jurisdiction or Target Area: Rhode Island

Primary Actor: Rhode Island Department of Health

Secondary Actor(s): N/A

Staffing utilized: No new staff was needed as part of this strategy. All program components, including the certification requirement and the information line, were integrated into departmental structures and staff time that already existed.

Other resources utilized: N/A

Factors essential to implementation: A law that required certification and training and a Department of Health committed to its implementation were key. A strong enforcement mechanism against those who do not use lead-safe work practices has been helpful.

Limitations/challenges/problems encountered: No significant problems or challenges were encountered in implementing this strategy, though many painters and remodelers continue to claim they aren't aware of the training requirements.

Magnitude of Impact/Potential Impact: Department of Health statistics show that 293 painters and remodelers have been trained through the lead-safe work practices requirements, and use of lead-safe work practices among target groups has increased since 1991.

Potential for replication: The potential for replication is high.

Contacts for Specific Information

Rosemary Aglione
Supervising Industrial Hygienist
Environmental Lead Program
Rhode Island Department of Health
401-222-7740
RosemaryA@doh.state.ri.us

Marie Stoeckel, CIH
Chief
Occupational Health Program
Rhode Island Department of Health
401-222-2438
MarieS@doh.state.ri.us

References for additional information

1. Rhode Island Lead Rules and Regulations
   www.rules.state.ri.us/rules/released/pdf/DOH/DOH_152_.pdf

TARGETING HIGH-RISK HOUSING

CAPITALIZE ON HOME NURSING VISITS TO TARGET PREVENTION SERVICES

CONNECT MEDICAID DATA AND STATEWIDE SURVEILLANCE DATABASES

CONSOLIDATE AND ANALYZE DATA TO HIGHLIGHT LEAD POISONING "HOT SPOTS"

EXTEND HOME ASSESSMENTS AND INTERVENTIONS FOR FAMILIES SERVED BY MEDICAID

PERFORM BUILDING-WIDE HAZARD ASSESSMENTS IN MULTI-UNIT BUILDINGS FOLLOWING IDENTIFICATION OF LEAD HAZARDS IN ONE TROUBLED UNIT

SCREEN HOMES DURING CODE INSPECTION

CAPITALIZE ON HOME NURSING VISITS TO TARGET PREVENTION SERVICES

DESCRIPTION OF THE STRATEGY

Visiting nurse programs offer a unique opportunity to efficiently reach pregnant women and new mothers in high-risk communities. Traditional home nursing visits can be enhanced to visually assess hazards, collect dust samples, inform occupants and rental property owners of hazards, demonstrate specialized cleaning methods for lead dust, and discuss lead poisoning risks. Further, and most critically, the nurses can provide referrals to available lead hazard control resources and other resources.

BENEFITS

Immediate/Direct Results: Education and referrals provided during home nursing visits directly benefit the families served. The physical presence of nurses in the homes provides a mechanism for nurses to identify conditions that may warrant emergency interventions, even outside the context of formal policies for such action.

Public Health Benefits: Lead safety improvements triggered by nurse visits benefit siblings and future occupants. In addition, home nurse visits provide a mechanism for targeting available lead hazard assessment and/or control services to high-risk families who can benefit immediately. Over time, cumulative efforts will help improve the lead safety of the housing stock.

Other Indirect/Collateral Benefits: Word-of-mouth among new mothers may reinforce efforts to raise awareness among families in the community. Nurse referrals may help generate referrals to other community programs, such as weatherization or lead hazard control, thereby reducing marketing efforts for such programs.

SCOPE OF POTENTIAL IMPACT

City- or County-Wide

PRIMARY ACTORS	**KEY PARTNERS**
Health Department	

CRITICAL ELEMENTS

Staff requirements: Staffing needs depend upon whether the lead activities are provided as an adjunct to home nurse visits that are already being made, or whether they are an entirely new service, and by the scope of services provided.

Other resource requirements: If nurses will be collecting dust samples or demonstrating lead-safe cleaning techniques, they will need the appropriate tools (such as wipes for dust sampling, HEPA vacuum, etc.) and protocols, along with any necessary training.

Institutional capacity required: Management support is the most likely element required for continued support of a staff-intensive effort.

Cost considerations: To maintain the visiting nurse program's existing coverage of its target population caseload, the incremental cost of adding lead safety to the visiting nurse protocol will need to be reimbursed so that the staff can be expanded accordingly.

Timing issues: Can be implemented at any time.

Feasibility of Implementation: High. As demonstrated by the adoption of this strategy in multiple jurisdictions, the strategy is feasible in multiple variations.

POTENTIAL OBSTACLES/BARRIERS

Use of this strategy requires ongoing commitment of nursing staff time and training.

If programs seek to add lead hazard education to previously planned nursing visits, they may run the risk of overwhelming both parents and the nurses by providing too much information at one time, ultimately making the sessions less effective.

Nurses and families may be frustrated by the lack of meaningful lead hazard control resources available in the community. Pregnant women may resist interventions that could lead to uncomfortable relationships with landlords or even evictions; the program should develop a contingency strategy for landlord retaliation (with assistance from a legal aid agency and/or the code enforcement agency) and explain it to their patients.

ADDITIONAL RESOURCES

N/A

ILLUSTRATION #1 OF STRATEGY IN PRACTICE

With the support of a CDC $100,000 primary prevention grant, WI CLPPP developed and pilot-tested a nursing home visitation program in two high-risk Wisconsin communities (Racine and Sheboygan). Although the one-time CDC grant has ended, the program since has evolved into a different but sustainable format, with 34 programs run by local health departments throughout the state.

The initial pilot program, which targeted low-income, primarily Medicaid-eligible, pregnant women through the Prenatal Care Coordination Program (PNCC), provided prenatal lead education and referrals, environmental assessments, and feedback to property owners. Fourteen PNCC nurses were trained as Lead Sampling Technicians and equipped with HEPA Vacuums. During initial prenatal home visits, a nurse provided information about childhood lead poisoning and potential lead hazards in the home environment. The nurse also conducted a visual assessment of the home, collected pre- and post-cleaning lead dust samples from floors and windows, demonstrated lead dust reduction measures, and provided cleaning supplies to the parent. During a second visit four-six weeks later, nurses reinforced messages and collected lead dust samples from the same locations to assess the effectiveness of measures that were taken to reduce lead dust. Pre- and post-cleaning results were provided to clients. Finally, property owners were informed in writing of the results of the dust sampling, given a copy of the HUD Lead-Paint Safety Field Guide, and encouraged to repair deteriorated painted surfaces. Families and property owners were also encouraged to enroll their properties in the HUD Lead Hazard Reduction Program if appropriate.

After CDC funding ended, Wisconsin revised the program to reach a broader target audience by adding an additional lead-specific home visit to existing prenatal and newborn visitation programs. Local health departments (LHD) now choose the level of intensity of services provided during their lead visits, selecting various combinations of three options: lead education, environmental assessments, and feedback to property owners. Due to capacity and resource constraints, not all LHDs are doing dust sampling; some are using LeadCheck swabs. The state is continuing to support local efforts, currently devoting about 15 percent of two FTEs to support the program and budgeting about $35,000 per year. Local LHDs estimate their costs at about $3,000 per year. To help build capacity and support dust sampling, Wisconsin is training an additional 23 nurses as lead sampling technicians and plans to offer free dust sample analysis through the state lab.

Jurisdiction or Target Area: Wisconsin

Primary Actor: WI Department of Health and Family Services, Childhood Lead Poisoning Prevention Program

Secondary Actor(s): Local health departments throughout the state

Staffing utilized: At the state level, the project required 0.2 FTE for the first year.

Other resources utilized: N/A

Factors essential to implementation: The willingness of visiting nurse program to train nurses as LSTs, and lab resources for dust wipe analysis, were essential to implementing this strategy.

Limitations/challenges/problems encountered: Initial concerns about creating conflict by contacting property owners proved to be mostly unfounded. In fact, the program has been so popular that nurses in one locality fought successfully to protect it from threatened budget cuts.

Magnitude of Impact/Potential Impact: During the nine-month pilot, approximately 100 families received services. WI CLPPP estimates that some level of service has been provided to about 500 families statewide this year, and expects the number to reach 1,200 by the end of year. The program has been well received statewide by nurses and families.

Potential for replication: High. Widely replicable in jurisdictions with visiting nurse programs.

Contacts for Specific Information

Sue LaFlash
Public Health Nurse
WI Childhood Lead Poisoning Prevention Program
608-266-8176
laflasi@dhfs.state.wi.us

Reghan Walsh
Health Education Specialist
WI Childhood Lead Poisoning Prevention Program
608-261- 9432
walshro@dhfs.state.wi.us

References for additional information
WI CLPPP has various program documents available in either hard copy or electronic form upon request. The core resource is the Prenatal and Newborn Home Visitation Resource Pack, which was designed specifically for local health departments to customize as needed. Also available is a Prenatal Education/Assessment Protocol.

ILLUSTRATION #2 OF STRATEGY IN PRACTICE

"Keep Your Baby Lead-Safe" ("KYBLS") is an innovative home visiting program developed by the RI CLPPP to educate pregnant women about lead hazards and connect them with resources to control lead hazards in their homes. Originally piloted in Providence, KYBLS is now a collaboration of the CLPPP, the Family Outreach Program (FOP), the Department of Administration's Energy Office, Blackstone Valley Community Action Project, and the Lead Hazard Reduction programs in the cities of Woonsocket and Pawtucket. Women eligible for KYBLS must both be pregnant and residing in either Woonsocket or Pawtucket; they may be either tenants or homeowners. Once enrolled, women receive an initial home visit from an FOP nurse (home visiting agency) who explains the project, administers an educational questionnaire on childhood lead poisoning, and answers any questions or concerns. With the family's authorization, the FOP nurse arranges a joint second visit with the Energy Office Weatherization Program to conduct a visual assessment of the property. Depending on the visual assessment and other conditions of the home and type of occupancy, the Weatherization Program may provide educational materials; refer to community resources; provide cleaning supplies and demonstrate cleaning techniques that help maintain a lead-safe home; collect lead dust wipe samples at both initial and final stages of the project (which are analyzed by the state laboratory); and, upon eligibility, help secure weatherization services and/or reduced-cost lead hazard reduction work.

Through partnership with the Weatherization program, the KYBLS project aims to literally get a "foot in the door" by delivering an energy-efficient, lead-safe environment at no cost and with minimal involvement of the property owner. Weatherization program policies do not require the permission of the property owner to perform an initial energy assessment. The property owner's signature is only needed in order to perform energy conservation treatments (which involve no cost to the property owner and no threat of legal penalty). CLPPP sought to utilize these facets of the Weatherization Program to initiate contact with property owners offering an opportunity to improve their properties for free, easing the concerns of women who feared conflict with or eviction by their landlord, and following up with contact regarding the need to repair lead hazards.

Following the birth of each participant's child, the program uses RI health department (KIDSNET) and CLPPP databases to identify and track the child up to the first blood lead level screen, to serve as another method of evaluation method for the project. The educational impacts of the KYBLS project continue to be assessed through an analysis of both the pre- and post- educational surveys administered to participants at the initial and final stages of their enrollment, as well as the pre- and post- dust wipe samples taken by the FOP workers at the homes of KYBLS enrollees. RI CLPPP has budgeted $100,000 per year for KYBLS.

Jurisdiction or Target Area: Rhode Island

Primary Actor: RI Department of Health Childhood Lead Poisoning Prevention Program

Secondary Actor(s): N/A

Staffing utilized: 0.75-1.0 FTE is supporting the project.

Other resources utilized: N/A

Factors essential to implementation: The essential factor is the cooperation between the health department and the weatherization agency.

Limitations/challenges/problems encountered: Unfortunately, implementation has proven to be very challenging, since a waiting list for weatherization services delays access to the property improvements to be provided at no cost, and property owners are not very enthusiastic about financing lead hazard controls via the loans that are offered. Many of the referred women refused services, could not be located, or did not meet eligibility requirements. Because the program began as a small pilot program, to date only a handful of properties have been successfully enrolled into lead hazard control or weatherization programs.

Magnitude of Impact/Potential Impact: From Nov. 2002 – Dec. 2003, 437 referrals were received, 135 women have been enrolled and received services, and another 52 women are being contacted to offer services.

Potential for Replication: Moderate if experience shows ways to overcome challenges encountered to date.

Contacts for Specific Information

Magaly Angeloni
Program Coordinator
Childhood Lead Poisoning Prevention Program
Rhode Island Department of Health
401-222-4602
magalya@doh.state.ri.us

Jill Barber
"KYBLS" Coordinator
Childhood Lead Poisoning Prevention Program
Rhode Island Department of Health
401-222-5932
JillianB@doh.state.ri.us

References for additional information
RI CLPPP is willing to share its educational brochures, protocols, and database design for KYBLS.

CONNECT MEDICAID DATA
AND STATEWIDE SURVEILLANCE DATABASES

DESCRIPTION OF THE STRATEGY

By linking the state's Medicaid data electronically with statewide lead poisoning surveillance databases, states determine testing rates for children served by Medicaid and identify children in the Medicaid caseload who have not been screened. Analysis of these data can also be used to identify and target neighborhoods in which numerous Medicaid children have been poisoned in order to direct prevention resources to areas at highest risk. Since 1998, CDC has been encouraging states to make these connections by requiring lead poisoning prevention grantees to have a system for ongoing identification of Medicaid-eligible children in the surveillance system, preferably via performing automated data linkages or matches between surveillance and Medicaid enrollment data sets.

BENEFITS

Immediate/Direct Results: Data sharing improves the ability of the lead program and state Medicaid agency to systematically target prioritized primary prevention in high-risk neighborhoods.

Public Health Benefits: Data sharing combines information sources and it sheds enormous light on "high-risk" Medicaid populations, who can be targeted for primary prevention. Combining information sources also permits agencies to focus EBL screening efforts in neighborhoods where screening is required but not happening and better monitor both case-identification rates and the actual delivery of lead screening services, including the performance of individual Medicaid managed care plans and medical practices. It can also permit agencies to track follow-up care provided by local health departments and justify Medicaid reimbursement for such services.

Other Indirect/Collateral Benefits: In addition to links between lead surveillance and Medicaid enrollment data, linkages can be established with other systems, such as geographic information system (GIS) coding and other programs' enrollment data. When illuminated by GIS, the matched data can yield clear and persuasive maps presenting risk, screening, or case-identification data for specific neighborhoods. The lead program can share analyses of the resultant combined data (suppressing identifying information) with housing agencies to facilitate targeting of resources for housing rehab and up-front lead hazard control to highest-risk blocks and block groups, or combine it with WIC enrollment data to discover risk relationships that can improve targeting strategies for primary or secondary prevention initiatives.

SCOPE OF POTENTIAL IMPACT

Statewide   City- or County-Wide

PRIMARY ACTORS	KEY PARTNERS
Health Department	Medicaid Agency

CRITICAL ELEMENTS

Staff requirements: Staffing needs depend on the status of the existing databases and the quality of the data therein. If the databases contain complete and accurate data, linkages can be made relatively simply through electronic means. For example, a 0.25 FTE can execute a concerted data matching and evaluation project linking and analyzing lead surveillance, Medicaid, and WIC data within one year. However, considerable staff time may be required if the data sets are incomplete or error-filled.

Other resource requirements: Investment in database software or hardware could be required to manage the upgrade of either data set and/or matching the data sets.

Institutional capacity required: Information system managers for both agencies must understand the project goals and have top-down support for a joint project. Interagency agreements and even legislation supportive of sharing the data may be required.

Cost considerations: Net costs depend on the status of the existing data systems. The cost of data matching is an allowable state administrative cost under Medicaid and therefore partially reimbursable by CMS.

Timing issues: Can be implemented whenever systems and support are in place.

Feasibility of Implementation: Very high. Implementation has been successfully implemented by 28 states, according to CDC: AK, AL, CA, CT, DE, FL, IA, IL, KS, LA, MD, ME, MI, MN, MO, NC, NH, NJ, OH, OK, OR, RI, TX, UT, VA, VT, WI, WY.

POTENTIAL OBSTACLES/BARRIERS

Poor quality underlying data is a prohibitive barrier to a successful data sharing project, as any data linkages are only as good as the information being compared. A common obstacle arises if the necessary data sets are housed in different agencies or in different locations, or split between agencies with poor working relationships. There is ample evidence that such obstacles can be overcome in any state, by enlisting senior management's early support for the project.

Privacy and confidentiality issues make all public agencies anxious about sharing data, and such concerns have been heightened by perceived new requirements associated with the Health Insurance Portability and Accountability Act's Standards for Privacy of Individually Identifiable Health Information (commonly known as the HIPAA Privacy Rule). It is imperative that proponents of data sharing be familiar with the facts about HIPAA as well as applicable state or local privacy policies. Some states have laws that require sharing of such data.

ADDITIONAL RESOURCES

A number of resources are available to assist states in taking this step. These include:

1. HCFA/HRSA/CDC Data Sharing Letter (10/22/98)
   www.cms.hhs.gov/states/letters/smd10228.asp
2. HCFA *Lead Screening* Letter to State Medicaid Directors (10/22/99)
   www.cms.gov/states/letters/smdo2299.asp
3. *The Foundations of Better Lead Screening for Children in Medicaid: Data Systems and Collaboration*, Alliance For Healthy Homes (formerly The Alliance To End Childhood Lead Poisoning), (April 2001)
   www.afhh.org/res/res_pubs/foundations.htm
4. CDC, *Working with Medicaid: a Resource Guide for Childhood Lead Poisoning Prevention Programs* (2001) (available on request from CDC Lead Branch)
5. CDC, *Surveillance for Elevated Blood Lead Levels Among Children — United States, 1997—2001*, MMWR Surveillance Summaries, September 12, 2003 / 52(SS10);1-21
   www.cdc.gov/mmwr/preview/mmwrhtml/ss5210a1.htm
6. Because of the central importance of the strategy to targeting efforts for lead screening, and thus to CDC, a number of case studies have already described implementation of this strategy in considerable detail. Detailed accounts can be found of the data-linking approaches, challenges, and results in the following states:

In the *Foundations* report (the more recent reference):

- North Carolina
- Oregon
- Wisconsin

In CDC's *Working with Medicaid* Resource book:

- Connecticut
- Iowa
- Illinois
- Missouri
- North Carolina
- Ohio
- Wisconsin

ILLUSTRATION OF STRATEGY IN PRACTICE

The Chicago CLPPP regularly matches its lead surveillance database with Medicaid eligibility and billing data (two separate Medicaid databases) to track and analyze screening and EBL rates. Each quarter, CLPPP performs a data match and then translates the results into a standardized report for the Medicaid agency. The report contains aggregate information on the number of Medicaid-enrolled children tested by age, race, address, and other factors of interest, as well as information on blood lead levels by various criteria. It also includes a list of untested children, which is used for direct outreach by CLPPP to encourage testing. In addition, since the data are geo-coded by address, the CLPPP program uses the data to validate high-risk areas for HUD funds and other prevention efforts and to generate "good visuals" (i.e., mapped data) that help in mobilizing partnerships for prevention in problem areas.

Jurisdiction or Target Area: Chicago

Primary Actor: Childhood Lead Poisoning Prevention Program (CLPPP) at the Chicago Department of Public Health (DPH)

Secondary Actor(s): Illinois Department of Public Aid

Staffing utilized: Developing the report takes one day of staff time.

Other resources utilized: N/A

Factors essential to implementation: The city health department successfully negotiated its data-sharing agreement directly with the state Medicaid agency, the Illinois Department of Public Aid. Program staff believes that the key ingredient for a successful project is the existence of a clean blood lead surveillance database, which can be a challenge given that it is constructed by the CLPPP from information provided by providers who collected the samples and the laboratories that analyzed the samples. In contrast, Medicaid data tends to be relatively clean. Chicago modeled its approach after two states' successful efforts (NC and WI). Chicago CLPPP staff sought advice and technical assistance from peers in those states, who were gracious about sharing their data matching protocols.

Limitations/problems/challenges: Completing development of the agreement between the agencies was regarded as the biggest challenge to the program.

Magnitude of Impact/Potential Impact: The data match and subsequent analysis have helped the Chicago CLPPP characterize the nature of two health care utilization gaps and to develop strategies to overcome them: children who have not presented for any well-child care and those who have sought care but still did not receive lead screening.

Potential for replication: High

Contacts for Specific Information

Anne Evens
Director, CLPPP, Chicago DPH
312-746-7824
evens_anne@cdph.org

Patrick MacRoy
Epidemiologist, CLPPP, Chicago DPH
312-746-5007
Macroy_Patrick@cdph.org

References for additional information
N/A

CONSOLIDATE AND ANALYZE DATA TO HIGHLIGHT LEAD POISONING "HOT SPOTS"

DESCRIPTION OF THE STRATEGY

Examining lead risk factors by geographic location allows for the identification of local variations in lead risk factors and provides an effective vehicle for communicating the presence of risk factors specific to a certain area. Geographic Information Systems (GIS), computer software capable of spatial analysis, permits powerful consolidation and analysis of multiple risk factors. GIS can be used to analyze address-specific data from various sources, including, but not limited to, Census data, local tax assessor and other housing data, blood lead surveillance data, and code violation data. With the encouragement and support of CDC, a number of CLPPP programs and researchers have employed GIS technologies to analyze lead risk data, present information powerfully, and develop more precise targeting strategies. GIS can also assist health departments, housing agencies, and others to focus lead hazard control and lead screening planning and can help such programs in allocating resources.

BENEFITS

Immediate/Direct Results: Use of GIS software allows spatial analysis of address-specific data, identifying high-risk geographic areas that may be difficult to discern by scanning lists or data sets. The software automates the labor-intensive process of manually mapping information, accommodates updates and additions to the data, and permits customization of analysis.

Public Health Benefits: Well-done analyses can yield more sophisticated and efficient targeting strategies for both primary and secondary prevention activities. They can also effectively illustrate situations where a single property is associated with repeated EBL cases and track properties that have been evaluated, renovated, or abated over time. Sometimes such analysis yields unexpected information such as clustering of cases, shedding light on previously unrecognized point sources or risk factors.

Other Indirect/Collateral Benefits: GIS analysis can yield data-driven findings that provide the scientific basis for motivating action by public officials. Indeed, computerized analysis of address-based data can counteract perceptions of bias about expected outcomes.

SCOPE OF POTENTIAL IMPACT

Statewide

City- or County-Wide

Regional (e.g. multi-county)

Neighborhood/Community

PRIMARY ACTOR

Health Department

KEY PARTNERS

Housing Agency

Property Taxation Agency

Human Services Agency

CRITICAL ELEMENTS

Staff requirements: Varies according to scope of project and existing capacity.

Other resource requirements: The quality of the existing databases is crucial: information must be complete and accurate. Correctly spelled addresses must be expressed in the same formatting conventions and terms that geo-coding programs recognize. Also, access to information technology expertise, software, and technical support.

Institutional capacity required: Securing access to the desired data may require programs to negotiate new data-handling agreements or take special programming steps to comply with privacy policies, especially with respect to the identity of children in lead surveillance databases, and in some circumstances, address information.

Cost considerations: There are out-of-pocket costs associated with programming, acquiring data, cleaning databases (if necessary), and licensing software; however, specific costs will vary depending on a number of factors. Purchase of GIS software is now an authorized expenditure for CDC CLPP grant funds.

Timing issues: Can be implemented at any time.

Feasibility of Implementation: Moderate. A number of programs have already deployed GIS technology successfully to analyze data related to lead poisoning prevention, providing useful models and resources for support, advice, and practical tools.

POTENTIAL OBSTACLES/BARRIERS

Although "mapping" feels approachable, the concept of Geographic Information Systems (GIS) can be intimidating for those unfamiliar with the software. Programs need to set clear goals for their analyses and decide if simple and focused will accomplish their goals (e.g., Wisconsin illustration), or if something more complex and comprehensive is appropriate (e.g., NCHH illustration).

A potential barrier that can require considerable staff time to remedy is the quality of the databases. Generally speaking, tax assessor databases are relatively clean, due to their importance to local government finances, while lead surveillance data tends to require cleaning to render it intelligible for GIS programs.

It is also possible that very small scale mapping (e.g., at the block level) of EBL data could trigger privacy concerns, so agencies must have clear policies in place in comply with prevailing privacy requirements.

ADDITIONAL RESOURCES

1. Kim D, Forrest S, Curtis GB, Buchanan S. *Relation Between Housing Age, Housing Value, and Childhood Blood Lead Levels in Children in Jefferson County, Kentucky, Using Geographic Information System Technology.* American Journal of Public Health, June 2002, 92(5):769-70.

2. Miranda, ML, Dolinoy, DC, and MA Overstreet. Mapping for Prevention: GIS Models for Directing Childhood Lead Poisoning Prevention Programs. Environmental Health Perspectives, Volume 110, Number 9, September 2002.

3. Reissman DB, Staley F, Curtis GB, Kaufmann RB. *Use of Geographic Information System Technology To Facilitate Health Department Decision-Making Regarding Childhood Lead Poisoning Prevention Activities.* Environmental Health Perspectives, Volume 109, Number 1, January 2001.

4. Roberts JR, Curtis GB, Hulsey T, Reigart JR. *Using Geographic Information Systems to Assess Risk for Elevated Blood Lead Levels in Children.* Public Health Rep 2003 118:221-229.

5. CDC staff have developed a white paper providing guidance on potential issues associated with the use of surveillance system address data. The paper, called *Preparing Surveillance Data for GIS Use* (January 2004), is available upon request to CDC's Childhood Lead Poisoning Prevention branch.

6. *The Foundations of Better Lead Screening for Children in Medicaid: Data Systems and Collaboration*, Alliance For Healthy Homes (formerly The Alliance To End Childhood Lead Poisoning), (April 2001). This report contains a case study describing Oregon's experience with GIS analysis of Medicaid-related data.
www.afhh.org/res/res_pubs/foundations.htm

ILLUSTRATION #1 OF STRATEGY IN PRACTICE

WI CLPPP used GIS software to produce maps demonstrating visually the association between childhood lead poisoning and age of housing. Specifically, Wisconsin developed a series of maps showing both the geographic location of residences of children with elevated blood lead levels (data from the state's blood lead surveillance system) and age of housing (data from US Census).

Jurisdiction or Target Area: Wisconsin

Primary Actor: WI Department of Health and Family Services, Childhood Lead Poisoning Prevention Program

Secondary Actor(s): N/A

Staffing utilized: Producing the maps required about 1 month of 1 FTE's time from the CLPPP. The CLPPP was able to tap into the State's Business Information Systems office to secure the expertise needed to create the data source files and deploy the GIS software (ArcView); this support required one month of 1 FTE in-kind.

Other resources utilized: N/A

Factors essential to implementation: The program partially credits the success of the maps to careful planning and testing to ensure that the messages were clear for the desired audiences. To this end, WI CLPPP pilot-tested the materials with nurses, health educators, and sanitarians from local health departments' lead program staff. The state is currently exploring the feasibility of offering online access to GIS mapping, through which the public would be able to customize maps of lead data in combination with various other types of data.

Limitations/challenges/problems encountered: None mentioned.

Magnitude of Impact/Potential Impact: Wisconsin created maps with 3 views for all of its 72 counties and the larger cities, enabling them to show separately the areas with low (0 – 30 percent pre-1950 housing), medium (30 – 60 percent), and high (60 – 100 percent) densities of older housing. The resulting maps were powerful communication tools showing strongly that those with lead poisoning are predominately found in the areas with the highest proportion of pre-1950 housing.

Although the maps were relatively straightforward in the sense that they only mapped one familiar risk factor (age of housing), feedback on the maps has been universally positive, with continuing requests for customization. At least one jurisdiction used them to target properties for HUD lead hazard control funding, and the city-level maps positioned cities for collaboration and communication about the use of Community Development Block Grant (CDBG) funds for prevention. Even private managed care organizations have requested detailed maps for their service areas, as they reportedly do not have GIS capability themselves. An unsolicited feedback letter from an insurance company requesting additional maps commented that they "*were a real visual learning experience for our head Pediatrician and, interestingly, … his nurse [said] they are now doing lead testing at 12 and 24 month [well child] visits. So the visual is a real WOW to nonbelievers.*"

Potential for replication: Moderate

Contact for Specific Information
Reghan Walsh
Health Education Specialist
WI Childhood Lead Poisoning Prevention Program
608-261-5817
walshro@dhfs.state.wi.us

References for additional information
WI CLPPP has various program documents available in either hard copy or electronic form upon request, including project descriptions and sample maps.

ILLUSTRATION #2 OF STRATEGY IN PRACTICE

In March 2002, the U.S. Department of Housing and Urban Development (HUD) contracted with the National Center for Healthy Housing (NCHH) to develop an interactive, web-based lead database that utilizes "real time" information and mapping capabilities to display housing and blood lead information related to lead hazards. NCHH has partnered with Abt Associates in Cambridge, Massachusetts to do the technical development of the database system and website. As part of HUD's strategy to eliminate childhood lead poisoning by 2010, this system is a demonstration project for other jurisdictions interested in using their local data in a similar way.

The website provides visitors with a number of choices of data sources and presentation modes. For example, visitors can view maps of EBL data by neighborhood, or lead or code violation data for a specific address, and plot lead risk factors by zip code, census tract, or other geographic areas. The system is designed to allow user to interface seamlessly with multiple local databases to target at-risk properties for services and education as well as enforcement activities. The system could also assist individual renters and buyers in identifying lead-safe or at-risk housing.

Jurisdiction or Target Area: Nationwide; pilot tested in Baltimore, Boston, and Chicago

Primary Actor: National Center for Healthy Housing, with Abt Associates

Secondary Actor(s): N/A

Staffing utilized: The pilot project has required an average of 1 FTE at each site, plus 4 FTEs at the national level, to develop the prototypes for these unique systems.

Other resources utilized: The pilot project was funded through a $3.5 million grant from HUD. Current funding will support the site through 2004. The project partners are currently seeking Federal, state, and private funds for ongoing support of the system. Estimates for the development costs for local jurisdictions to replicate and maintain the approach are expected to be well below the costs of initial development. Costs to replicate the system will be affected by local characteristics, including: quality and "cleanliness" of the existing blood lead surveillance, housing, and other relevant data sets willingness and ability of local governments to share property-level information, and technical capacity of the jurisdiction with respect to GIS readiness (e.g., availability of "shape" files).

Factors essential to implementation: NCHH and Abt Associates consulted with stakeholders in each of the three cities to determine what data should be included in the database; how that data will be collected, cleaned, and incorporated in the database system; and how it will be maintained over time. Stakeholders included local and state health and housing agencies, community groups and advocates, health care providers, nonprofit housing organizations, and others. As a result, six key features were selected: "real time" health and housing data; one location for health and housing data; housing data at the address level; health data at a higher level of aggregation; mapping capabilities; and links to other websites containing useful information.

Limitations/problems/challenges: Overcoming concerns of property owners, the local real estate industry, and the health department over privacy issues required problem solving. As a consequence, all blood lead data is aggregated at the block group level and is not viewable for specific addresses. And, if fewer than 25 children are included, then the blood lead data is not displayed at all.

Magnitude of Impact/Potential Impact: The project has been piloted in Baltimore, Boston, and Chicago. Comprehensive, "real time," address-specific data is a distinguishing feature. Address-level information will help localities focus their efforts and target resources toward the areas of greatest need.

Potential for Replication: Moderate. The conceptual and technical development supported by HUD's pilot project can greatly facilitate local replication if the resources to sustain and accurately update the information systems are in place at the local level. Cost estimates for replicating the approach are forthcoming.

Contacts for Specific Information

Rebecca Morley
Executive Director
National Center for Healthy Housing
410-992-0712
RMorley@centerforhealthyhousing.org

Pat McLaine
Assistant Director for Program Management
National Center for Healthy Housing
410-992-0712
PMcLaine@centerforhealthyhousing.org

References for additional information
1. www.LeadSafeHomes.info

EXTEND HOME ASSESSMENTS AND EARLY INTERVENTIONS FOR FAMILIES SERVED BY MEDICAID

DESCRIPTION OF THE STRATEGY

Through collaboration between government agencies and community groups, a comprehensive set of environmental and educational services are provided to Medicaid families whose child has been identified with a blood lead level that is moderately elevated. Services include in-home lead education, risk assessment, lead hazard control, and post-work clearance sampling. All families with an EBL child and the owners of any rental units occupied by them receive a written plan with specific recommendations for hazard control and help in identifying financial assistance and getting training in lead-safe work practices. On an as-needed basis, the program provides to eligible households free lead hazard reduction measures that vary from abatement to low-level interim controls, such as window repair or replacement, paint stabilization, grass seeding, cleaning, and paint maintenance plans.

BENEFITS

Immediate/Direct Results: Children with moderately elevated blood lead levels (e.g. in the 10 to 19 μg/dl range) receive individual environmental and educational services that are provided in many jurisdictions only to children with higher blood levels, providing them with better prospects for improved outcomes. The program's focus on lead hazard reduction is an important benefit for Medicaid families who might otherwise only receive educational or medical interventions.

Public Health Benefits: The strategy bridges the gap between primary and secondary prevention by protecting children before poisoning occurs and preventing exposure to children occupying the same housing in future years. Focusing interventions on Medicaid families exemplifies the kind of risk-based targeting recommended by CDC and HUD.

Other Indirect/Collateral Benefits: By repairing lead hazards in the homes of Medicaid families, the program contributes to the development of a lead-safe housing stock for low-income families in the community over time.

SCOPE OF POTENTIAL IMPACT

Specific/Targeted Population—Resource-intensive interventions impact target group of families

PRIMARY ACTORS	KEY PARTNERS
Department of Social Services	Health Department
Housing Agency	Economic and Community Development Agencies
	Community-based Organizations
	Medical Centers
	Code Inspection Agency

CRITICAL ELEMENTS

Staff requirements: Staffing needs vary depending on the scope of the project. For example, a pilot project serving a limited community and 52 families required 1 FTE.

Other resource requirements: N/A

Institutional capacity required: Effectively providing seamless services to targeted families requires having mechanisms in place to secure referrals from health care providers, health departments, and others who may identify Medicaid families eligible for services. Adequate means for complying with medical privacy requirements must also be in place. Program staff, partners, or contractors must have the appropriate expertise and training and any applicable credentials to provide lead education services, hazard determination, and lead hazard control services.

Cost considerations: Such intensive service delivery can be expensive: $300-400 for a risk assessment, $500-20,000 for lead hazard control, $150 for a clearance examination. Federal Medicaid policies allow reimbursement for environmental investigation and case management services. However, at present some state Medicaid programs have not begun reimbursing for these services despite explicit federal encouragement to do so. Lead hazard control can be funded by a variety of sources.

Timing issues: Program could be implemented whenever resources, referral mechanisms, regulatory compliance measures, and service providers have been secured.

Feasibility of Implementation: Moderate. This is an ambitious program requiring strong community commitment, significant resources, and ongoing collaboration among disparate entities. Beginning with a pilot program is one means to establish relationships and test systems.

POTENTIAL OBSTACLES/BARRIERS

This project requires considerable coordination and cooperation between various agencies and entities including health, housing, and the state Medicaid agency. It would likely be difficult to acquire the resources and support for this type of project in a situation where adequate environmental responses are not available to families whose children have even higher blood lead elevations (above 20 μg/dL).

ADDITIONAL RESOURCES

N/A

ILLUSTRATION OF STRATEGY IN PRACTICE

Lead Action for Medicaid Primary Prevention (LAMPP) is sponsored by CT Department of Social Services, in partnership with CT Department of Public Health and CT Department of Economic and Community Development. LAMPP was developed by the CT Get The Lead Out Coalition (comprised of community and policy organizations) and is managed under contract by Connecticut Children's Medical Center with support from the Regional Lead Treatment Centers at Yale-New Haven and Hartford. LAMPP provides early intervention services to Medicaid children with blood lead elevations too low (below 20 μg/dL) to trigger state requirements for abatement and full case management services. The program's goal is to prevent further rises in BLL and more serious damage to children.

Jurisdiction or Target Area: Connecticut

Primary Actor: CT Department of Social Services

Secondary Actor(s): CT Department of Public Health and CT Department of Economic and Community Development

Staffing utilized: The pilot project required 1 FTE. The expanded program now underway requires a total of 6.3 FTEs, including project director, project coordinator, relocation coordinator/educator, administrative/clerical assistant, social work supervisor, and a construction supervisor.

Other resources utilized: LAMPP was launched originally as a pilot project funded by the state health department for $200,000 focused on providing lead education and risk assessments, with limited ability to fund lead hazard control. After about 18 months' experience assisting 52 families, LAMPP secured two grants totaling $5.6 million from HUD's Office of Healthy Homes and Lead Hazard Control. Matching contributions from partner communities exceed $5 million dollars in in-kind health education, housing code enforcement, and housing rehabilitation assistance.

Factors essential to implementation: The tenacity of the Get the Lead Out Coalition in promoting the project and the willingness of the project partners to work collaboratively were essential.

Limitations/challenges/problems encountered: This initiative is limited to properties occupied by Medicaid families with young children or pregnant women, and targeted to eleven Connecticut cities with large numbers of Medicaid enrolled children but limited or no funding for lead hazard control.

Magnitude of Impact/Potential Impact: LAMPP accepts referrals from medical care providers, local health departments, courts, and others, and provides families with education and risk assessments, individualized plans for reducing lead hazards, and low-level housing interventions. Under the expanded program, which began Oct. 1, 2003, LAMPP provides lead-safe work practices training for landlords who do their own maintenance work, for remodeling, painting, and maintenance personnel, and for volunteer groups such as Christmas in April. LAMPP expects to create lead-safe environments for children in 562 housing units (interim controls and standard treatments in 433 units, and more intensive lead hazard abatement in 129 more units) over 42 months. With a goal of collecting future Medicaid reimbursements for eligible services, the LAMPP program has positioned itself by affiliating with the agency that administers Connecticut's Medicaid program (Social Services).

Potential for replication: Moderate

Contact for Specific Information

Ronald Kraatz
LAMPP Project Director
Connecticut Children's Medical Center
860-545-9602
RKraatz@ccmckids.org

David Parrella
Director
Medical Care Administration
Connecticut Department of Social Services
860-424-5978
David.Parrella@po.state.ct.us

References for additional information
N/A

PERFORM BUILDING-WIDE HAZARD ASSESSMENTS IN MULTI-UNIT BUILDINGS FOLLOWING IDENTIFICATION OF LEAD HAZARDS IN ONE TROUBLED UNIT

DESCRIPTION OF THE STRATEGY

If lead hazards are identified in one unit in a multi-family building (through an EBL investigation or other means), there is a significant likelihood that similar hazards may be present in other units in the building due to common painting and maintenance histories. Undertaking building-wide hazard assessments in multi-unit buildings (complemented by building-wide blood lead screening of other young children who are occupants, especially if there was an elevated blood lead level already detected) is a useful strategy for targeting high-risk units. Agencies could extend this approach to screen all properties owned or managed by the same person or entity, especially "problem landlords."

BENEFITS

Immediate/Direct Results: Environmental assessments triggered in this manner can benefit other children who reside in the same property before they might be exposed to lead or by identifying current, but previously unrecognized, lead hazards earlier than they might otherwise have been.

Public Health Benefits: This strategy efficiently targets limited public health inspection resources to properties and families that are predictably at higher risk.

Other Indirect/Collateral Benefits: Consistent application of this strategy raises awareness of lead hazards and reinforces messages about their relationship to housing.

SCOPE OF POTENTIAL IMPACT

Statewide City- or County-Wide
Neighborhood/Community

PRIMARY ACTORS
Housing Agency

KEY PARTNERS
Health Department
Code Inspection Agency
Human Services/Medicaid Agency

CRITICAL ELEMENTS

Staff requirements: An agency must provide sufficient staff to oversee property referrals and handle necessary administrative responsibilities. Hazard assessment capacity could be acquired by hiring staff or by contracting with private service providers.

Other resource requirements: N/A

Institutional capacity required: Authorization to enter properties and share data as needed.

Cost considerations: Systematically screening other units in the same building where one has hazards can be a cost-effective primary prevention strategy.

Timing issues: None

Feasibility of Implementation: Moderate feasibility

POTENTIAL OBSTACLES/BARRIERS

The experience of the Massachusetts Department of Public Health (DPH) is illustrative of some difficulties associated with this strategy. While its regulations authorize the health department to conduct building-wide investigations, the agency does not routinely do so because of concern that generating multiple orders for correction of hazards will divert the owner's resources from addressing the unit that has poisoned a child. As an alternative, DPH notifies all tenants in a building about an inspection, advising that lead was found in one unit, it is likely that their unit has lead, and they should talk to the owner or call the state or local board of health if they want an inspection. Upon tenant request, DPH does an investigation. Additionally, DPH will investigate other units in those jurisdictions where local financing agencies in Massachusetts will assist owners with abatement of all units in the building at once. Massachusetts is revisiting its strategy for multi-unit buildings as it develops its CDC-required strategic plan.

ADDITIONAL RESOURCES

N/A

ILLUSTRATION OF STRATEGY IN PRACTICE

Maine law and regulations require the Department of Human Services to inspect all units in a building occupied by a lead-poisoned child and perform an environmental investigation in all units that (1) have visible potential lead hazards, and (2) are occupied by a child under age six. The inspection report and, if applicable, an order to abate identified lead hazards within 30 days are provided to property owners. Typically, public health nurses conduct informal outreach to parents in the building or arrange for a group education session to encourage building-wide blood lead level screening.

Jurisdiction or Target Area: Maine

Primary Actor: Maine Department of Health and Human Services

Secondary Actor(s): N/A

Staffing utilized: Maine DHS dedicates one FTE to coordination and oversight of the CLPP environmental program, including assuring the required inspections of multi-family properties. To access inspectors on an "as needed" basis, Maine DHS contracts with five Community Action Agencies and two private inspector firms.

Other resources utilized: N/A

Factors essential to implementation: Maine DHS has patched together the necessary funds from multiple sources, including Medicaid reimbursement for investigation of properties occupied by eligible lead-poisoned children, funds from the state's maternal and child health block grant, and reimbursement for inspection if the property owner enrolls in the HUD-funded Lead Hazard Control grant program, by the Maine State Housing Agency or city government that receives HUD LHC grants.

Limitations/challenges/problems encountered: Securing the resources to pay for environmental investigations has been the biggest challenge. Although not a common problem, inspections occasionally create conflict between landlords and tenants. Although Maine law specifies that a household cannot be evicted due to a child's lead poisoning, Maine is considering strengthening tenant protections against landlord retaliation.

Magnitude of Impact/Potential Impact: Program staff estimate that 250 multi-family buildings have been investigated after the identification of a lead-poisoned child in one of the units since the 1999 law was enacted.

Potential for replication: High.

Building Blocks for Primary Prevention: Protecting Children from Lead-Based Paint Hazards

Targeting High-Risk Housing

PERFORM BUILDING-WIDE HAZARD ASSESSMENTS IN MULTI-UNIT BUILDINGS FOLLOWING IDENTIFICATION OF LEAD HAZARDS IN ONE TROUBLED UNIT

Contact for Specific Information

Mary Ann Amrich

Program Manager, CLPPP

Department of Human Services

207-287-8753

maryann.amrich@state.me.us

References for additional information

1. State law authorizing building-wide environmental investigations is available in Chapter 252—The Lead Poisoning Control Act. See §1320-A "Inspection of dwellings by department"
   http://janus.state.me.us/legis/statutes/22/title22ch0sec0.html

2. December 2003 agency rules codifying program requirements
   ftp://ftp.state.me.us/pub/sos/cec/rcn/apa/10/144/144c292.doc

3. The Maine CLPPP is willing to share its detailed protocols for environmental investigations, including detailed requirements for inspection reports.

SCREEN HOMES DURING CODE INSPECTION

DESCRIPTION OF THE STRATEGY

Code inspections prompted by complaints about housing problems such as a roof leak, roaches, or no heat, as well as routine periodic inspections of rental housing units, provide opportunities to screen for lead hazards and peeling paint in the homes of young children. Code enforcement staff can be specially trained to conduct limited checks for lead hazards as a means to trigger additional action. If the inspection identifies a lead hazard through visual assessment, spot testing, dust testing, or paint testing, the inspector can order the property owner to undertake lead hazard control or lead-safe repair work to bring the unit into compliance with any applicable standards.

BENEFITS

Immediate/Direct Results: The number of homes checked for lead hazards can be greatly increased at comparatively low cost by integrating basic lead safety checks into other code inspection visits. By checking homes for lead hazards and requiring corrective action consistent with applicable standards, code enforcement programs help reduce the risk of childhood lead poisoning.

Public Health Benefits: In most jurisdictions, the lead poisoning prevention program sends environmental investigators only to the homes of children who have been lead poisoned. In contrast, code inspectors have the opportunity to enter many homes, and they can identify hazards before a child is exposed and an elevated blood lead level develops. Their code enforcement authority can be used to routinely intervene to require lead safety in the highest risk older properties—those that are subject to tenant complaints about poor maintenance or other health conditions.

Other Indirect/Collateral Benefits: This approach leverages limited public inspection resources to trigger lead hazard assessment control. Strong enforcement broadens impact of the code enforcement program, prompting property owners to undertake voluntary measures in other properties and perform preventive maintenance on all rental housing.

SCOPE OF POTENTIAL IMPACT

City- or County-Wide

PRIMARY ACTORS

Code or Building Inspection Agency

KEY PARTNERS

Health Department
Local Prosecutors
Property Owners
Contractors

CRITICAL ELEMENTS

Staff requirements: During the start-up phase of a statewide program, approximately 0.75 FTE is needed to establish procedures and build trained capacity. For an established program, 0.3 FTE is needed for program oversight and one FTE for technical assistance to local agencies (code agency and health department). For local agencies, each individual who conducts housing inspections should be trained to perform lead determinations. Depending on the sampling method used, checking for lead hazards will add 10-30 minutes to the typical housing inspection. Staff requirements to meet the workload will depend on the type of determination, which is affected by what the standard is: no peeling or otherwise non-intact paint in any housing, no lead dust hazards, etc. Depending on the extent of lead hazards, the standard to be met, the type of enforcement action, and the local or state court rules, additional time is also required for enforcement steps, including court appearances. Inspectors represent themselves at hearings before clerk magistrates or judges, as they already do for other code enforcement cases. Involvement of public agency attorneys is generally needed only for cases that progress to the criminal complaint stage.

Other resource requirements: Supplies or equipment to check paint; supplies and lab services to check dust.

Institutional capacity required: This strategy requires authority to require compliance with an explicit standard (e.g. no peeling or otherwise non-intact paint in any housing, no plumbing leaks, no lead dust hazards), such as statutory lead safety requirements for housing or locally adopted property maintenance code. The statutory authority should cover licensing or certification of code inspectors or categorically exempt trained inspectors employed by public agencies from licensing or certification requirements. Implementation needs include training curricula, and, as needed, training providers approved by an accreditation program to teach the curriculum. Continuing partnership between agencies that regulate lead-based paint activities and those that enforce codes will ensure effective implementation.

Cost considerations: The program will be more effective if resources are available to assist low-income property owners with the cost of lead hazard control and provide favorable financing terms to others.

Timing issues: Can be implemented whenever infrastructure is in place.

Feasibility of Implementation: Moderate. In jurisdictions that have code enforcement apparatus and enforceable lead safety standards, this can be implemented wherever political will is sufficient to support enforcement. Enforcement can include requiring interim lead hazard controls rather than full lead hazard abatement, so as to decrease costs of compliance when code violations are found.

POTENTIAL OBSTACLES/BARRIERS
Lack of legal authority and absence of enforcement standards can be insurmountable barriers. Enforcement includes a single brief inspection and may involve multiple court appearances by the inspector to trigger and complete the legal process of enforcement. Two potential obstacles are the unwillingness of the city/county attorney to prosecute cases and the difficulty agencies may face in maintaining a presence in court throughout the entire enforcement process. State health departments could loan lawyers to prosecute and/or provide technical assistance to local agencies on request.

ADDITIONAL RESOURCES
N/A

ILLUSTRATION OF STRATEGY IN PRACTICE
Code enforcement staff who respond to complaints about housing problems such as a roof leak, roaches, or no heat, as well as routine periodic inspections of rental housing units are specially trained to conduct limited checks for lead hazards as a means to trigger additional action. If the inspection identifies a lead hazard through visual assessment, spot testing, dust testing, or paint testing, the inspector orders the rental property owner to undertake lead hazard control or lead-safe repair work to bring the unit into compliance with any applicable standards.

Jurisdiction or Target Area: Massachusetts

Primary Actor: Department of Public Health, Childhood Lead Poisoning Prevention Program

Secondary Actor(s): N/A

Staffing utilized: During the start-up phase, approximately 0.75 FTE was needed to establish procedures and build trained capacity. The established statewide program needs 0.3 FTE for program oversight and 1 FTE for technical assistance to local agencies (code agency and health department). Including this function in the responsibility of local housing inspectors reduces the number of inspections by a small increment. The inspector must acquire a special license for code enforcement lead determination inspectors; prerequisites for the license include employment by a code enforcement agency or local board of health, completion of the CLPPP training course, passing the licensing exam, and completion of a field apprenticeship.

Other resources utilized: N/A

Factors essential to implementation: Program staff in MA found the following factors to be especially critical to implementation:
1. The underlying statutory structure authorizing standards, licensing, and enforcement;
2. Implementation plans that were developed in collaborative fashion through an advisory committee (Governors Advisory Committee) with local health departments to ensure that procedures would be workable for them;
3. An inexpensive lead screening technique (sodium sulfide testing) that makes the program accessible to all localities in state; and
4. Continuous support of enforcement structure, beginning with advance notice to courts that enforcement cases would begin appearing.

Limitations/problems encountered: Program staff found that the most significant limitation was the lack of resources for lead hazard control. Despite longstanding Lead Law requirements, enhanced enforcement when the lead determination program was launched made it seem like a new requirement to property owners. Program staff feel that it was important to be able to offer resources to property owners to help with financing of lead work since the principal defense offered by property owners is that they don't have the money to abate. Consequently, the state has made available several different resources, including a state deleading tax credit, the "Get the Lead Out" revolving loan fund (originally funded through state appropriation but now primarily from repayments of prior loans), CDBG funds, and now a lower cost, moderate-risk do-it-yourself option for property owners. This last option involves training property owners in the use of lead-safe work practices to allow them to control moderate-risk lead hazards without the need for certified contractors.

Magnitude of Impact/Potential Impact: Since most lead determinations and subsequent enforcement actions occur at the local level and a statewide database is under development, the state lacks complete knowledge of the impact to date. The state provides lead determination services when local capacity is lacking or on special request (e.g., local government is property owner). For FY03, seven state inspectors did 150 lead determinations upon parental request, resulting in 85 homes undergoing lead hazard control.

Potential for replication: Moderate

Contact for Specific Information
Paul Hunter
Director of Childhood Lead Poisoning Prevention Programs
617-624-5757
Paul.Hunter@state.ma.us

References for additional information

1. S. 460:700: Enforcement by Code Enforcement Agencies
   www.state.ma.us/dph/clppp/1054601.pdf

2. Division of Community Sanitation
   www.state.ma.us/dph/dcs

USING CODE ENFORCEMENT AND OTHER SYSTEMS

ABATE LEAD HAZARDS AND RECOVER COSTS WHEN OWNERS FAIL TO ACT

ATTACH PROPERTY-SPECIFIC LEAD HAZARD INFORMATION TO PROPERTY DEEDS

COMPILE STATE AND LOCAL LAWS TO EXPEDITE LEAD SAFETY

CONDUCT PERIODIC HOUSING CODE INSPECTIONS

CONSOLIDATE CHILDHOOD LEAD POISONING PREVENTION AND CODE ENFORCEMENT ACTIVITIES

CREATE A SPECIAL LEAD COURT

ENABLE TENANTS AND COMMUNITY-BASED ORGANIZATIONS TO TAKE ACTION TO ADDRESS SUBSTANDARD HOUSING CONDITIONS

EQUIP CODE OFFICIALS TO IDENTIFY LEAD HAZARDS AND PURSUE ENFORCEMENT

INFORM RENTAL PROPERTY OWNERS OF FEDERAL LEAD HAZARD DISCLOSURE REQUIREMENTS

PRECLUDE OWNERS FROM RENTING UNITS THAT HAVE BEEN CITED FOR HAZARDS

REPORT PROBLEM RENTAL PROPERTY OWNERS TO HUD AND EPA FOR DISCLOSURE ENFORCEMENT

REQUIRE AGENCIES TO DISSEMINATE LEAD POISONING PREVENTION INFORMATION

REQUIRE AN INSPECTION FOR LEAD-BASED PAINT HAZARDS AT TENANT TURNOVER

REQUIRE RENTAL PROPERTY REGISTRATION/LICENSING

UTILIZE EARLY WARNING SYSTEMS FOR DETERIORATING PROPERTIES

ABATE LEAD HAZARDS AND
RECOVER COSTS WHEN OWNERS FAIL TO ACT

DESCRIPTION OF THE STRATEGY

Strong enforcement powers and sufficient resources to compel compliance are essential to any effective lead poisoning prevention program. In order to ensure that lead hazards cited by violation orders are controlled when property owners fail to act, enforcement officials can be authorized to abate hazards using agency or contractors' crews and recoup the costs along with any unpaid penalties by placing a lien on the property.

BENEFITS

Immediate/Direct Results: Homes containing lead hazards are immediately made lead-safe.
Public Health Benefits: The cycle of poisoning, where one unit poisons multiple children, is stopped.
Other Indirect/Collateral Benefits: Since the agency is carrying out or overseeing the work, it is more likely to be done correctly and without harming current occupants.

SCOPE OF POTENTIAL IMPACT

Statewide   Regional (e.g. multi-county)
City- or County-Wide   Neighborhood/Community

PRIMARY ACTORS

Health Department
Code or Building Inspection Agency
Local prosecutors

KEY PARTNERS

Housing Agency

CRITICAL ELEMENTS

Staff requirements: Limited to writing lead hazard control work specifications, ensuring acceptable completion including clearance, and administrative communications to collect costs or impose lien.

Other resource requirements: Access to qualified crews, contracted or in-house, to perform the lead hazard control.

Institutional capacity required: Agencies will need statutory authority to enter the premises and do the work, as well as to place a lien on the property. In addition, the agency will need capacity to perform independent clearance testing.

Cost considerations: Need for working capital or other financing to pay for the repair work pending recovery of costs when the property is sold or refinanced.

Timing issues: None.

Feasibility of Implementation: Moderate. Political will is needed to supersede owners' rights, to allow the city or its agents authority to enter the property and perform lead hazard control, and to impose liens. Strategy is best used within a continuum of approaches that include voluntary compliance and financing mechanisms.

POTENTIAL OBSTACLES/BARRIERS

May require relocation of occupants; these costs would be included in the owner indebtedness to the city.

ADDITIONAL RESOURCES

N/A

ILLUSTRATION OF THE STRATEGY IN PRACTICE

Title 6 of the Philadelphia Code and Regulations gives the Department of Public Health (DPH) the authority to issue correction orders to owners (or their agents) of housing units found to have lead-based paint hazards. If an owner does not comply with the order, the City files a case in Philadelphia's special "lead court." The city may seek a range of remedies, including the use of City funds to abate the hazard and recovery of those costs from the owner. If the property owner fails to reimburse the city, the court may place a lien on the subject property for the amount of abatement costs and other related expenses. This process has been a powerful motivator for property owners, who are now more likely to proactively correct lead hazards—or at least comply with orders before the case gets to court.

Jurisdiction or Target Area: Philadelphia, PA

Primary Actor: City of Philadelphia Law Department, Health and Adult Services Unit

Secondary Actor(s): N/A

Staffing utilized: There are no staff dedicated to implementing this strategy. When abatement is needed, crews from the city's lead hazard control program can be assigned and the labor cost is included in the amount billed to the property owner or added to the lien.

Other resources utilized: The Department of Health provides justification for the cases, including lead inspection checklists and laboratory records on EBLs. The Law Department also has access to a list of property owners who have requested assistance.

Factors essential to implementation: The combination of a dedicated lead court, consistent enforcement, and outreach to landlords to make sure they understand that they must comply or they will be prosecuted enables the City to avoid using this strategy.

Limitations/challenges/problems encountered: The City is unlikely to recover the costs of lead hazard control because homes with deferred maintenance and serious hazards, which often already have tax liabilities or other liens attached, sell for as low as five to ten thousand dollars. As a result, this measure is used only when owners qualify for no other programs. Also, determining the identity of the property owner is sometimes challenging and takes a considerable amount of time.

Magnitude of Impact/Potential Impact: The provision has not been used because the Law Department has been able to use other means to resolve the 1,700 cases that it has filed with the Court.

Potential for Replication: High.

Contacts for Specific Information

Lynda Moore
Chief Deputy, Health and Adult Services
215-683-5137
lynda.moore@phila.gov

Richard Tobin
Director, Childhood Lead Poisoning Prevention Program
215-685-2788
richard.tobin@phila.gov

References for additional information
N/A

ATTACH PROPERTY-SPECIFIC LEAD HAZARD INFORMATION TO PROPERTY DEEDS

DESCRIPTION OF THE STRATEGY

The federal lead hazard disclosure law requires property owners to communicate the presence of known lead-based paint and lead hazards to the prospective buyer or tenant when selling or renting a property built before 1978. However, disclosure requirements are not consistently implemented or understood. As a result, buyers may purchase properties without knowledge of existing and identified lead hazards. To ensure that buyers are informed of these lead hazards, copies of lead hazard violations, repair orders, and clearance reports could be attached to the property deed and available for review through the title search. Attaching property-specific lead hazard information to the deed would also offer the potential to monitor future disclosure of the identified hazards to prospective and renewal tenants in the property.

BENEFITS

Immediate/Direct Results: Documented hazards alert prospective purchasers and tenants to hazards. If prospective purchasers are unwilling to purchase properties with existing lead hazards and bear the cost of repair, property owners may be motivated to remediate hazards.

Public Health Benefits: Properties that have already been identified as sources of potential or actual poisoning receive attention. As a result, future occupants with young children will be living in a lead-safe environment.

Other Indirect/Collateral Benefits: Attaching property-specific lead hazard information to the deed allows the public agency to track and document owner knowledge of lead hazards. This public record could be used to verify compliance with disclosure requirements and bolster enforcement, thereby ensuring that a greater number of new or renewal rental tenants receive disclosure.

SCOPE OF POTENTIAL IMPACT

Statewide

PRIMARY ACTORS

Code or Building Inspection Agency
Housing Agency
Property Taxation Agency

KEY PARTNERS

Registry of Deeds

CRITICAL ELEMENTS

Staff requirements: No additional full-time staff is required to successfully enact this strategy. Implementation requires only the cooperation of existing Registry of Deeds staff.

Other resource requirements: N/A

Institutional capacity required: The federal disclosure law requires property owners to divulge known information about lead-based paint and lead hazards. The Registry of Deeds must be given the authority to attach lead hazard violations, repair orders, and clearance reports to individual property deeds. Statutory authority to issue code violations on lead hazards (and/or standards for issuing orders to reduce identified lead hazards) increases the impact of the disclosure law.

Cost considerations: Attachment to title involves the cost to process the appropriate paperwork. Using the illustration below, the average cost is $24 per order (based on one charge for the first page and a lower charge for each additional page). The charge varies based on the length of the order.

Timing issues: None.

Feasibility of Implementation: Very high. With no new funding, training programs, staff members, or equipment required, this strategy is easy to implement and should be viable in most jurisdictions.

POTENTIAL OBSTACLES/BARRIERS

The Registry of Deeds must have the statutory authority to attach orders to the deed, so jurisdictions interested in implementing this strategy should check current regulations and advocate for the appropriate changes. Another consideration is ensuring that confidential information related to any associated blood lead tests taken during the identification of the hazards is handled appropriately.

ADDITIONAL RESOURCES

N/A

ILLUSTRATION OF STRATEGY IN PRACTICE

If a lead investigation reveals an existing or potential lead exposure hazard, the State issues an Order of Lead Hazard Reduction (order) on the property, which requires that all lead exposure hazards be corrected. Under federal law, property owners are required to disclose the presence of lead hazards when selling or renting a property, but owners do not always comply. To ensure that buyers are aware of an outstanding order, the New Hampshire Childhood Lead Poisoning Prevention Program (NHCLPPP) sends all orders to the Registry of Deeds, which then attaches the order to the property deed. In the event that the owner attempts to sell the property without proper disclosure, the purchasers will discover the order during the routine title search.

Jurisdiction or Target Area: New Hampshire

Primary Actor: New Hampshire Department of Health and Human Services, Office of Community and Public Health, Childhood Lead Poisoning Prevention Program.

Secondary Actor(s): N/A

Staffing utilized: No additional staffing was required. The only additional effort required is printing a second original order and obtaining a signature from the NHCLPPP director.

Other resources utilized: N/A

Factors essential to implementation: The Registry of Deeds must have the authority to attach lead hazard violations, repair orders, and clearance reports to individual property deeds.

Limitations/challenges/problems encountered: This is an indirect strategy that strengthens the federal disclosure law and helps ensure that buyers are aware of untested lead hazards.

Magnitude of Impact/Potential Impact: NHCLPPP expects the attachment to increase the number of properties coming into compliance over time, as owners will be motivated to remediate hazards in order to sell the property.

Potential for replication: Very high. NHCLPPP has found this to be simple, low-cost strategy to implement.

Contacts for Specific Information

Michelle Dembiec
Program Manager
603-271-4507
mdembiec@dhhs.state.nh.us
leadinfo@dhhs.state.nh.us

Kathi L. Guay
Register of Deeds, Merrimack County
603-228-0101
kguay@aol.com

References for additional information

1. N.H. Code Admin. R. Ann. He-P 1602.34 (2001) (defines "order of lead hazard reduction")
   www.gencourt.state.nh.us/rules/he-p1600.html
2. N.H. Code Admin. R. Ann. He-P 1612.03 (2001) (proscribes that all orders of lead hazard reduction shall be recorded with the Registry of Deeds for the county in which the property is situated)
   www.gencourt.state.nh.us/rules/he-p1600.html

COMPILE STATE AND LOCAL LAWS TO EXPEDITE LEAD SAFETY

DESCRIPTION OF THE STRATEGY

State and local jurisdictions can help expedite primary prevention of childhood lead poisoning by disseminating applicable statutes and regulations in a user-friendly reference resource. Effective compilations include information about the full range of local, state, and federal lead poisoning prevention laws and regulations, including those governing lead-safe work practices, lead hazard control, rental property maintenance, and housing code requirements and enforcement mechanisms. This material can be researched, produced, and updated by entities such as health or housing agencies, court system agencies, law schools, or legal services programs. The compilations can take many forms, including bench books for attorneys and judges, and binders for use by health and code enforcement departments, community-based organizations, and property management companies.

BENEFITS

Immediate/Direct Results: State and local agencies and courts will be able to expedite lead safety in homes and apartment buildings when all relevant laws and regulations are easily accessible.

Public Health Benefits: Another tool will be added to assist state and local jurisdictions stop a cycle where housing units repeatedly poison children.

Other Indirect/Collateral Benefits: Statutory and regulatory compilations can make agencies and courts more efficient, saving time, resources, and taxpayer dollars.

SCOPE OF POTENTIAL IMPACT

Statewide   City- or County-wide

PRIMARY ACTORS	KEY PARTNERS
Health Department	Judges
Housing Agency	Local prosecutors
Code or Building Inspection Agency	Other attorneys
	Landlords
	Law schools/legal services
	Community-based organizations

CRITICAL ELEMENTS

Staff requirements: Initial compilation of documents can require 50 to 100 hours from an attorney or legal assistant. Maintaining and updating the documents may require nominal time after any policy change is enacted.

Other resource requirements: Access to paper and electronic copies of applicable state and local statutes and regulations is critical. Agencies also require search tools to locate these statutes and regulations.

Institutional capacity required: The agency producing the compilation needs staff familiar with state and local lead poisoning prevention laws and regulations. A legal intern could be valuable for this work.

Cost considerations: Excluding staff salaries and printing costs, this strategy should be cost effective. Limiting the number of printed copies by making the compilation available online or through e-mail in PDF format can reduce costs.

Timing issues: None.

Feasibility of Implementation: High.

POTENTIAL OBSTACLES/BARRIERS

There are two potential obstacles to this strategy's success. First, if case law is desired in the compilation, search tools are needed to locate past cases on lead poisoning prevention. Second, staff or interns may lack the time to maintain and update the compilation.

ADDITIONAL RESOURCES

N/A

ILLUSTRATION OF THE STRATEGY IN PRACTICE

In August 2004, Loyola University of Chicago School of Law presented to the Cook County Housing Court bench book on lead paint poisoning to assist the court in lead hazard control orders and taking other steps to help the county and the City of Chicago prevent childhood lead poisoning. The bench book explains the lead poisoning problem in Chicago and Cook County. It also provides a comprehensive set of lead laws for Chicago and Illinois, lead poisoning prevention case law in Illinois, and important reference appendices.

Jurisdiction or Target Area: Cook County, IL, including Chicago

Primary Actors: Loyola University of Chicago School of Law; Cook County Housing Court

Secondary Actor(s): N/A

Staffing utilized: 1 FTE (mostly interns) for one to one and a half months.

Other resources utilized: Appendix information came from various state and federal agencies, and the Corporation Counsel's office reviewed the bench book for accuracy and completeness.

Factors essential to implementation: It was essential to find up-to-date information, and to present that information verbatim. The information had to be summarized in an objective, non-judgmental manner to help judges apply the law independent of subjective information and anecdotes, and to allow judges and attorneys to be as efficient as possible by consistently consulting the same edition of lead poisoning prevention and safety laws.

Limitations/challenges/problems encountered: There were no significant limitations or challenges producing the bench book for Cook County. However, as Loyola tried to develop bench books for other counties in Illinois, it found it difficult to: a) to understand the court procedures in some of the other counties; b) identify who could provide information on the procedures and the information included in the Cook County bench book appendix; and c) identify the appropriate people to discuss distribution of the bench books.

Magnitude of Impact/Potential Impact: Unknown.

Potential for Replication: High.

Contacts for Specific Information

Anita Weinberg
Clinical Professor and Director, ChildLaw Policy Institute
Loyola University of Chicago School of Law
312-915-6482
aweinbe@luc.edu

References for additional information

N/A

CONDUCT PERIODIC HOUSING CODE INSPECTIONS

DESCRIPTION OF THE STRATEGY

Code enforcement systems that operate solely in response to tenant complaints, although the prevailing norm nationwide, are highly ineffective and have limited impact. This approach fosters the decline of rental housing conditions since tenants may not know how to register complaints or may be reluctant to complain out of fear of retaliation by the landlord. In contrast to sole reliance on complaint-based approaches, proactive, periodic inspection programs can advance primary prevention more meaningfully. Both New Jersey and Los Angeles have committed to inspecting multi-family rental properties every three to five years. Such preemptive code inspections also can be more narrowly targeted to high-risk neighborhoods, as the City of Milwaukee is doing.

BENEFITS

Immediate/Direct Results: Problems such as lead hazards are routinely identified by an inspection, documented, and brought to the attention of the rental property owner. Code officials can ensure that when housing code violations are corrected, the work is done in a lead-safe manner.

Public Health Benefits: A periodic rental housing inspection program helps to ensure that multi-family rental housing units comply with basic health and safety standards. Periodic inspections foster pro-active maintenance because property owners cannot expect to remain "outside the system." By promoting routine preventative maintenance on a widespread basis and improving the quality of the rental housing stock, periodic inspection programs can help to prevent lead hazards—even in rental housing units that would be missed under a complaint-based inspection program.

Other Indirect/Collateral Benefits: Periodic inspection programs, when coupled with an effective enforcement regimen, can generate fees sufficient to offset the cost of the program. Regular inspections help to maintain the quality of the rental housing stock over the long term in a cost-effective manner.

SCOPE OF POTENTIAL IMPACT

Statewide—Impact depends upon the scope of the housing code inspection program
City- or County-Wide
Neighborhood/Community

PRIMARY ACTORS	KEY PARTNERS
Code or Building Inspection Agency	Health Department
	Local Prosecutors
	Community-based Organizations
	Property Owners
	Tenants

CRITICAL ELEMENTS

Staff requirements: When moving from a complaint-based inspection program to a periodic system, additional inspectors may initially be required because a periodic inspection program also must accommodate complaints. Under an effective periodic inspection program, the number of complaint-based inspections will decrease over time. Where periodic inspections have been mandated, few inspections are undertaken in response to complaints. In New Jersey, for example, periodic inspections have been mandated for over thirty years, and few inspections currently are undertaken in response to complaints. Under the state's periodic inspection program, approximately 115 inspectors conduct approximately 162,000 inspections in dwelling units annually and re-inspect about 127,000 of those units.

Other resource requirements: As additional code inspectors are employed, they must be provided essential equipment and technical support, including vehicles and computers.

Institutional capacity required: Statutory authority is required in order to give housing code inspectors authority to enter rental housing to conduct regular inspections. Statutes should specify the universe of units to be inspected (e.g., rental housing in buildings with two or more units); how frequently inspections are to be conducted; what type of notice is required for each party (owner and tenant); funding sources for inspections (e.g., any fees imposed upon rental property owners to cover inspection costs); and enforcement provisions, including penalties for non-compliance. Newly hired inspectors will need to be qualified to conduct inspections, issue notices of violation, and commence enforcement actions. Experienced inspectors will require continuing education to ensure that they are aware of any new standards or technological advances.

Cost considerations: Even if the costs of periodic inspections are passed along directly to tenants, these programs need not have an adverse effect on affordable housing. When Los Angeles adopted its Systematic Code Enforcement Program in 1998, the city hired 67 new housing inspectors. The program was initially funded by a $1.00 per unit fee each month, which since has been increased to $2.27. New Jersey uses a sliding scale to determine the per-unit inspection fee imposed upon owners, dependent upon the number of units inspected. The maximum per-unit fee is $43 every five years.

Timing issues: Hiring and training of additional inspectors may take several months. In addition, landlords will need to be made aware of the new requirements, will need to receive guidance in building improvement requirements, and will need to incorporate periodic inspection language into leases. Tenants will also need education on the new requirements and procedures.

Feasibility of Implementation: High. These programs are feasible and effective, assuming they are adequately funded and enforced.

POTENTIAL OBSTACLES/BARRIERS

Perhaps the greatest obstacle facing periodic inspection programs is generating the political will necessary to put the programs in place.

ADDITIONAL RESOURCES

1. City of Milwaukee
   Department of Neighborhood Services Administration
   841 N. Broadway Room 104
   Milwaukee, WI 53202
   414-286-3441

ILLUSTRATION #1 OF STRATEGY IN PRACTICE

Under Los Angeles' Systematic Code Enforcement Program (SCEP), adopted in 1998, every residential rental property with two or more units must be inspected on a regular basis (currently, units are inspected at least once every five years). The program was funded initially by a $1.00 per unit per month fee paid by property owners, which, under the law, can be passed on to tenants. Low-income tenants strongly supported the passage of the program, including the monthly fee, which since has been increased to $2.27. Los Angeles is in the process of incorporating lead hazard screening into its periodic inspections, including requiring lead-safe work practices when repairs are undertaken. To complement the SCEP, a loan program has been created to provide funds to small apartment owners to help them finance repairs.

Jurisdiction or Target Area: Los Angeles

Primary Actor: Los Angeles Housing Department, Code Enforcement Bureau

Secondary Actor(s): The city has worked very closely with community-based organizations (CBOs) and advocates for affordable housing and lead poisoning prevention to ensure the effectiveness of the program.

Staffing utilized: More than 57 inspectors devote their time solely to proactive inspections. An additional 22 inspectors respond to tenant complaints. Some of the inspectors that deal with complaints also assist with re-inspections in units found to be out of compliance during the scheduled inspections.

Other resources utilized: N/A

Factors essential to implementation: Successful implementation of a periodic inspection program requires, first and foremost, adequate staff to carry out inspections. Inspectors must be well trained, not only to identify code violations, but also to deal effectively with tenants. In Los Angeles, advocates have conducted trainings for inspectors to help them deal with cultural and/or language issues that may arise with tenants.

Another key to the success of the SCEP program is that a loan program has been put in place to help small landlords make repairs. Finally, effective enforcement is critical to the success of a periodic code inspection program. While the city experienced some initial problems with cases stalling in the courts, hearing officers are increasingly successful at moving cases forward. In addition to a commitment to enforcement on the part of agency staff, adequate prosecutorial resources must be dedicated to enforcement.

Limitations/challenges/problems encountered: Initially, obtaining funds for the program was a challenge. However, the City increased the monthly inspection fee that rental property owners pay.

Magnitude of Impact/Potential Impact: The current schedule for inspections allows for rental units to be inspected every five years. Each year, about 150,000 units are inspected. However, the city hopes to increase that figure to 180,000.

Potential for replication: Very high. These programs are readily replicated.

Contact for Specific Information:
Greg Spiegel
Staff Attorney
213-487-7211
gspiegel@wclp.org

References for additional information:
1. Los Angeles Municipal Code, Chapter XVI, Housing Regulations, § 161.351 *et seq.*
2. Los Angeles Housing Department website
   www.lacity.org/lahd/index.htm

ILLUSTRATION #2 OF STRATEGY IN PRACTICE

Multiple dwellings (defined to include buildings with three or more units), hotels, and motels are required under New Jersey's Hotel and Multiple Dwelling law to be inspected at least once every five years. The state imposes a per-unit inspection fee every five years upon owners according to a sliding scale, dependent upon the number of units to be inspected: $43 per unit for one to seven units; $27 for eight to 24 units; $23 for 25 to 48 units, and $16 for 49 units and up. The state also collects approximately $4 million annually in penalties, enough to cover the program's costs when combined with the inspection fees. New Jersey law gives the Department of Community Affairs authority to adjust the program's fees to cover the cost of the program. In January 2004, New Jersey's governor signed a law requiring periodic inspections to include checks for lead hazards.

Jurisdiction or Target Area: New Jersey

Primary Actor: Bureau of Housing Inspection (BHI), which is part of the Division of Codes and Standards in New Jersey's Department of Community Affairs (DCA).

Secondary Actor(s): N/A

Staffing utilized: The state employs 65 inspectors (FTEs) and approximately 150 municipal inspectors (FTEs) to conduct all inspections on behalf of the state. Municipalities are reimbursed for their inspection costs through a State-Local Cooperative Housing Inspection Program. Code inspectors must be licensed.

Other resources utilized: A computerized tracking system is required to track compliance and enforcement.

Factors essential to implementation:
1. Inspection fees and penalties for non-compliance must be sufficient to cover the costs of the inspection program.
2. A streamlined enforcement process minimizes the resources needed to ensure compliance:
   a. If an owner fails to contest a violation within 15 days of receiving a citation, the owner is deemed to admit to the violation.
   b. If the owner fails to remedy the violation in a timely manner, BHI imposes a penalty and sets a deadline for compliance.
   c. Owners who fail to comply and pay the penalty are pursued in court, where they are barred from contesting the violation.
   d. Once BHI obtains a judgment, it can impose a lien on the owner's assets—both personal and corporate.

Limitations/challenges/problems encountered: One limitation on New Jersey's program is that it does not address buildings with fewer than three dwelling units. Efforts have been underway to include those buildings in the periodic inspection program but have not succeeded to date.

Magnitude of Impact/Potential Impact: New Jersey's periodic inspection program inspects approximately 162,000 dwelling units per year, and over time, achieves compliance in 95% of cases.

Potential for replication: Very high. These programs are readily replicated and highly effective.

Contact for Specific Information
Amy Fenwick Frank
Section Chief, NJ DCA, Division of Codes and Standards
609-292-7899
afrank@dca.state.nj.us

References for additional information
1. New Jersey Hotel and Multiple Dwelling Law, N.J.S.A. § 55:13A-1 *et seq.*
2. New Jersey Administrative Code, § 5:10 *et seq.*
3. New Jersey Department of Community Affairs, Division of Codes and Standards
   www.state.nj.us/dca/codes/

CONSOLIDATE CHILDHOOD LEAD POISONING PREVENTION AND CODE ENFORCEMENT ACTIVITIES

DESCRIPTION OF THE STRATEGY

Co-locating the childhood lead poisoning prevention program (CLPPP) and the public agency responsible for housing and sanitation code enforcement is an option for local governments to facilitate collaboration between traditionally separate activities. An even stronger consolidation extends to the CLPPP authority to cite violations of the housing code's provisions related to deteriorated paint and lead hazards and trigger enforcement proceedings. In some instances, it may be preferable for the agencies to physically move closer or even share an office suite, but for other local governments, simply increasing collaboration can have significant results.

BENEFITS

Immediate/Direct Results: Co-locating CLPPPs with code enforcement agencies will expedite responses to the lead hazards by the code enforcement authority, helping CLPPPs bridge the gap between these functions that exists in many jurisdictions. When CLPPPs share code enforcement authority, or can influence its actions, they can readily ensure that owners of homes with deteriorated paint or other lead hazards identified by the CLPPP will be required to fix the hazards.

Public Health Benefits: Improved code enforcement is the cornerstone of primary prevention. CLPPP staff will be able to effectively prioritize enforcement to benefit the highest risk children and housing. As a result of increased awareness of lead hazards among code enforcement staff, routine code enforcement practices can evolve to recognize violations that may have previously been considered low priority, triggering violation notices that may not have been generated in the absence of an EBL child.

Other Indirect/Collateral Benefits: Improved code enforcement will lead to growth in the number of lead-safe or lead-free homes.

SCOPE OF POTENTIAL IMPACT

City- or County-Wide

PRIMARY ACTORS

Health Department
Housing Code or Inspection Agency

KEY PARTNERS

City/County Prosecutors

CRITICAL ELEMENTS

Staff requirements: Staff requirements depend upon agency responsibilities and resources. Where enforcement authority coexists, more staff is likely to lead to more citations.

Other resource requirements: Field staff expected to evaluate houses for lead hazards will need training, certification, and possibly an XRF device.

Institutional capacity required: To the extent that code enforcement authority is shared or delegated, legislative, regulatory, or executive agency action may be needed. Substantive cross-agency coordination and/or resource sharing require upper management support.

Cost considerations: Lab analysis costs ($50 per home on average), training, and prosecution resources associated with an incremental increase in the number of inspection staff and inspections performed. Certification costs for public employees are waived in some jurisdictions.

Timing issues: Can be implemented whenever administrative and management arrangements have been completed.

Feasibility of Implementation: High with management support.

POTENTIAL OBSTACLES/BARRIERS

The housing code enforcement agency may be reluctant to delegate authority to or share it with the CLPPP staff because they will not trust that the staff will follow the procedures properly. Staff may also be concerned about overwhelming the legal system needed to complete the enforcement process. If the housing code enforcement has been lax in the past, suddenly adding lead hazard enforcement will be controversial with property owners.

ADDITIONAL RESOURCES

N/A

ILLUSTRATION OF STRATEGY IN PRACTICE

When the city and the county consolidated operations in the mid-1970s, the health department and the county hospital became part of a quasi-governmental corporation. The county delegated responsibility for housing code enforcement to the health department and subsequently established an Environmental Court to prosecute housing code violations and related issues. The CLPPP issues citations for houses where it finds deteriorated paint or lead hazards, often as a result of an environmental investigation of a lead poisoned child. Between January 2000 and July 2003, the CLPPP issued more than 200 citations and pursued those cases in the Environmental Court to get the hazards resolved.

Jurisdiction or Target Area: Marion County / Indianapolis

Primary Actor: Childhood Lead Poisoning Prevention Program, Housing Division, Marion County Health Department, Marion County Health and Hospital Corporation (includes Indianapolis).

Secondary Actor(s): N/A

Staffing utilized: Six FTE staff trained and licensed as risk assessors conduct the inspections, manage the enforcement process, and re-inspect some properties as needed.

Other resources utilized: The close cooperation of the inspectors with other CLPPP staff enhances the overall effectiveness of the program. The Environmental Court streamlines the process and ensures that the hazards are addressed.

Factors essential to implementation: The agency responsible for housing code enforcement must be willing to cooperate with the CLPPP staff and have a streamlined process to enforce code citations.

Limitations/challenges/problems encountered: Staff must follow specific procedures and be prepared for the delays as property owners must be notified and prodded with orders and fines to address the problem.

Magnitude of Impact/Potential Impact: Between January 2000 and July 2003, the CLPPP issued more than 200 citations and managed those citations in the Environmental Court to get the hazards resolved.

Potential for replication: Very high

Contact for Specific Information
Dave McCormick
Director, CLPPP
317-221-2171
dmccormi@hhcorp.org

References for additional information

1. See www.mchd.com/newlead.htm for a description of CLPPP program.
2. See www.mchd.com/newlead.htm for a copy of the Residential Housing Code.

CREATE A SPECIAL LEAD COURT

DESCRIPTION OF THE STRATEGY
One obstacle to effective enforcement of lead safety in housing is the lack of enforcement capacity. Establishing a special lead court to focus the applicable court system's consistent attention on cases involving violations of lead hazard repair orders can reduce a backlog and enable the assigned judge(s) to become familiar with repeat violators and treat them accordingly. Philadelphia and Chicago have significantly accelerated the processing of cases and reduced the backlog of properties pending corrective action by dedicating court resources to these cases.

BENEFITS
Immediate/Direct Results: Outstanding orders to address lead hazards are enforced, lead hazards are repaired, and more housing comes into compliance more quickly.

Public Health Benefits: Repeat violators are identified and treated accordingly. Future residents are protected from lead poisoning.

Other Indirect/Collateral Benefits: Code enforcement is given the teeth it needs to be effective and the possibility of court action motivates property owners to become more proactive in eliminating lead hazards. Property Court case backlog is cleared, increasing the efficiency of the court system and freeing enforcement personnel to attend to new cases.

SCOPE OF POTENTIAL IMPACT
City- or County-Wide

PRIMARY ACTORS
City/County Solicitors and Prosecutors
Judges
Inspection, Code, or Building Agency

KEY PARTNERS

CRITICAL ELEMENTS
Staff requirements: The extent of staffing (lawyers and paralegals) must meet the needs of the enforcement caseload.

Other resource requirements: N/A

Institutional capacity required: Statute that allows city to hold property owners responsible for code violations is necessary to give the health department the authority to go after landlords. The Court must determine how to implement the court by reworking existing courtrooms and judge assignments.

Cost considerations: No additional cost if court is funded to fulfill its mandates.

Time issues: None

Feasibility of Implementation: High. This strategy could be successfully replicated where there exists a statute granting the jurisdiction to the inspection and enforcement authority and cooperation between the Court, the city prosecutor's office, and the inspection office exists. Other useful factors include lead hazard control funds to assist landlords with the repairs.

POTENTIAL OBSTACLES/BARRIERS

A big challenge is identifying the actual property owner. A rental property registration system identifying owners' names and contact information would overcome this problem.

ADDITIONAL RESOURCES

N/A

ILLUSTRATION OF STRATEGY IN PRACTICE

Three days a week, a special Lead Court convenes within Philadelphia's Court of Common Pleas to hear complaints regarding outstanding lead hazard orders; each session hears an average of 20 cases. City attorneys set forth all possible remedies available to the city under the various codes, including fines; relocation of tenants at the owner's expense; and if the owner fails to abate, abatement by the city with authorization to recover costs or place a lien on the property. The potential for court action acts as a great motivator: in the majority of cases, owners have begun the work prior to the hearing, and typically the court responds by ordering that the property owner complete the work by a specified deadline. In instances where the city has had to do the abatement work, the court works out payment plans with property owners to recoup the cost.

Jurisdiction or Target Area: Philadelphia

Primary Actor: City of Philadelphia Law Department; Court of Common Pleas; Department of Health's Inspections and Enforcement Division, Childhood Lead Poisoning Prevention Program.

Secondary Actor(s): N/A

Staffing utilized: One City-contracted attorney appears in court, and 2 FTE Law Department paralegals work on paperwork, filings, and other preparatory work.

Other resources utilized: N/A

Factors essential to implementation: Cooperation and communication between the Department of Health, the Law Department, and the Court are critical. It also requires outreach to property owners and community groups to educate them on lead poisoning, the law, and the lead court process. The Inspections and Enforcement Division also offers free training each month, which covers lead-safe work practices, personal protection procedures, the pros and cons of various lead hazard reduction methods, and the biological effects of exposure.

Limitations/challenges/problems encountered: The challenge that arises most often is the identification of a property's actual owner.

Magnitude of Impact/Potential Impact: When the lead court began in November 2002, a backlog of 1,426 cases existed. As of February 2004, the lead court had heard 943 cases. More than 650 orders have been completed. The City of Philadelphia has five times the compliance it had before the creation of the lead court.

Potential for replication: High. As long as the key public agencies are willing to make it happen, this could be replicated anywhere.

Contacts for Specific Information

Lynda Moore
Chief Deputy
Health and Adult Services
City of Philadelphia Law Department
215-683-5137
lynda.moore@phila.gov

Joseph Kauffman
Program Manager
Inspections & Enforcement
Philadelphia Department of Public Health
Childhood Lead Poisoning Prevention Program
215-685-2788
joseph.kauffman@phila.gov

References for additional information

N/A

ENABLE TENANTS AND COMMUNITY-BASED ORGANIZATIONS TO TAKE ACTION TO ADDRESS SUBSTANDARD HOUSING CONDITIONS

DESCRIPTION OF THE STRATEGY

In many cases, tenants lack the ability to address substandard housing conditions or are reluctant to exercise their rights out of concern that the landlord will retaliate. Empowering tenants to take action when housing conditions are inadequate and enabling neighborhood organizations to act on tenants' behalf can significantly enhance the efforts of code enforcement officials. One effective strategy is to legally enable tenants or their advocates to request a code inspection and empower them to pursue enforcement actions themselves in court. This approach also helps circumvent the common problem of inadequate resources for enforcement.

BENEFITS

Immediate/Direct Results: Tenants in substandard properties obtain legal standing to initiate code inspections, enforcement, and remediation actions without fear of landlord retaliation. If receiverships (court appointment of third party administrators to manage properties and oversee repairs) or rent escrow arrangements are permitted, rents can be used directly to fund repairs.

Public Health Benefits: High-risk housing is targeted for repairs that reduce health hazards. Code agency and/or court oversight can ensure that repairs are done safely and following accepted protocols and without hazards being left behind.

Other Indirect/Collateral Benefits: Tenants gain power in relation to landlords, which could result in landlords community-wide becoming more responsive and proactive regarding maintenance and repairs.

SCOPE OF POTENTIAL IMPACT

City- or County-Wide   Neighborhood/Community
Specific (Targeted) Population—Rental Housing

PRIMARY ACTORS

Community-based Organizations

KEY PARTNERS

Code or Building Inspection Agency
Housing Agency
Local Prosecutors
Property Owners
Tenants
Contractors
Painters

CRITICAL ELEMENTS

Staff requirements: An experienced organizer could, in several months, organize a campaign capable of enacting such a law. One or more FTE (organizers, attorneys) could staff a project to assist tenants with using the process in just one community. Enacting a new state or municipal law to give legal standing for tenants in substandard properties to initiate code inspections/enforcement and take enforcement actions themselves can be a major undertaking.

Other resource requirements: Research would be needed on existing laws, as well as on the degree and extent of substandard housing conditions in the jurisdiction and specific shortcomings of the existing code enforcement system.

Institutional capacity required: An organization undertaking such a campaign would need the capacity to organize and lobby, experienced staff, and relationships with allies among tenants' rights, affordable housing, public interest, legal, and other community organizations.

Cost considerations: The positive impact on housing affordability and condition is potentially great. These benefits will far exceed the cost of a campaign to secure enabling legislation. Creating and funding an organization or agency to provide ongoing assistance to tenants bringing enforcement cases should be considered, as this will greatly improve the impact of the law and the quality of outcomes.

Timing issues: None

Feasibility of Implementation: Variable. Any organization undertaking such an effort should understand that because of the complex and unpredictable nature of the legislative process, the degree of difficulty may be greater than expected and success is not guaranteed. Pilot programs with limited scope may be a useful first step, giving advocates time and resources to prove that the strategy is effective in a target area.

POTENTIAL OBSTACLES/BARRIERS

This strategy requires enacting new legislation, working to ensure that it is effectively implemented, and ongoing work to assist tenants with using the process. Thus, this strategy is a major undertaking and could fail if sufficient resources and energy are not available to overcome inertia and political opposition.

ADDITIONAL RESOURCES

N/A

ILLUSTRATION OF STRATEGY IN PRACTICE

Minnesota's landlord-tenant law, Chapter 504B, allows tenants, a municipality, or a neighborhood housing-related organization legal standing to bring a court action against a landlord who fails within a reasonable time to correct deficiencies at their property. Project 504, a non-profit neighborhood organization, has brought more than ten such cases in the past three years, leading to broad remedies for tenants, including in some cases the appointment of a third-party administrator to manage and operate the landlord's property. Project 504's court action also established precedent that significant unabated lead hazards in a property constitute an emergency, causing the court to issue orders to the landlord to correct the hazards immediately.

Jurisdiction or Target Area: Minnesota (Minneapolis)

Primary Actor: Project 504

Secondary Actor(s): N/A

Staffing utilized: Part-time involvement of a legal services attorney and a social worker/organizer.

Other resources utilized: Digital and video cameras, resources for meeting support, cell phones.

Factors essential to implementation: Strong partnership with other affordable housing and tenant advocacy organizations. Code enforcement officials who recognize that the strategy's success will reduce enforcement time spent on problematic properties. Strong and ongoing relationships with tenants, including any identified tenant leaders who will advance the strategy. Solid knowledge of landlord-tenant law, or partnership with *pro bono* or legal services attorney who can provide legal analysis and support. Relationships with proactive landlords who recognize the need to address substandard housing in their jurisdiction are also helpful.

Limitations/challenges/problems encountered: Language barriers should be expected and budgeted for in non-English speaking communities. Some code enforcers may view this strategy as infringing on their traditional role and turf. Strong initial negative reaction from some landlords should be expected, possibly followed by retaliation against the project or some tenants upon implementation.

Magnitude of Impact/Potential Impact: More than 200 families have directly benefited since 1999, with 200 additional units/families benefiting from the strategy's incidental effects on neighboring properties. Project 504's example has prompted the City of Minneapolis to pursue a similar strategy, leading to the filing of nearly 200 city-initiated cases since 2001.

Potential for Replication: Moderate.

Contact for Specific Information
Gregory Luce
Co-Director
612-221-3947
gluce@project504.org

References for additional information
1. www.project504.org
2. Minn. Stat. § 504B.395
   www.revisor.leg.state.mn.us/stats/504B/395.html
3. Documents available by request from Project 504

EQUIP CODE OFFICIALS TO IDENTIFY LEAD HAZARDS AND PURSUE ENFORCEMENT

DESCRIPTION OF THE STRATEGY

Because their mandate is to ensure that substandard housing conditions are identified and corrected, code enforcement officials are in an ideal position to prevent children from becoming poisoned. In addition, code officials routinely enter substandard properties prompted by other code violations. Training code officials to identify lead hazards and arming them with enforcement powers creates an opportunity for them to identify lead hazards and require action before children are poisoned. For example, code inspectors can take the one-day Lead Sampling Technician training to learn how to sample dust for lead hazards. Inspectors can also alert property owners to lead-safe work practices and resources for learning these.

BENEFITS

Immediate/Direct Results: Dwellings come into compliance with lead safety requirements, health hazards are reduced, decay and deterioration are minimized, and the appearance of buildings is substantially improved. Lead-burdened homes that repeatedly poison children can also be made safe through this strategy.

Public Health Benefits: The next occupant's children will be safe from lead hazards; decline in prevalence of lead poisoning.

Other Indirect/Collateral Benefits: Heightened community awareness about lead hazards and lead poisoning.

SCOPE OF POTENTIAL IMPACT

Regional (e.g. multi-county)
City- or County-Wide (The logical scale is the jurisdiction of the agency that is doing the inspections)

PRIMARY ACTORS

Code or Building Inspection Agency

KEY PARTNERS

Health Department
Housing Agency
Training Providers
Lead Hazard Control programs

CRITICAL ELEMENTS

Staff requirements: Beyond one-day training, there will be minimal impact on inspection staff to incorporate deteriorated paint into the inspection protocol. Additional staffing may be needed in the short term for repeat inspections to ensure compliance with repair orders.

Other resource requirements: N/A

Institutional capacity required: The jurisdiction's health, housing, or property maintenance code must provide the investigating department with enforcement authority.

Cost considerations: Jurisdictions with funding assistance for property owners may be more successful.

Timing issues: N/A.

Feasibility of Implementation: Moderate. Feasible where there is applicable code and a will to enforce it.

POTENTIAL OBSTACLES/BARRIERS

Landlords may resist making repairs citing cost considerations; the city must be prepared to enforce code requirements against recalcitrant owners and landlords.

ADDITIONAL RESOURCES
N/A

ILLUSTRATION #1 OF STRATEGY IN PRACTICE

Dubuque's housing inspection staff is responsible for licensing and inspection of the City's 7,500 rental properties. Rental properties are inspected on a five-year cycle; owner-occupied properties are inspected on a complaint-only basis. The inspection includes a visual inspection for loose, flaking, and/or chipping paint on either interior or exterior surfaces; deteriorated paint is cited as a code violation. Lead-based paint is assumed in pre-1978 properties. Owners/landlords are advised to use lead-safe work practices in repairing the paint. Follow-up inspections are made until the work is done. Noncompliant properties are posted and, in extreme cases, vacated until repairs are made. Handouts and other educational materials accompany the inspection process. The Department also trains owners, landlords, contractors, workers, and others on using lead-safe work practices in painting or renovations.

Jurisdiction or Target Area: Dubuque, Iowa

Primary Actor: Housing and Community Department

Secondary Actor(s): N/A

Staffing utilized: No information provided.

Other resources utilized: No information provided.

Factors essential to implementation: Dubuque is a very historic city, and there is a lot of pride in its appearance. There are also numerous incentives to make repairs, including the city's comprehensive rehabilitation program that offers financial assistance, its Operation Paint Brush (which helped many lower income homeowners paint their houses), and a Lead Hazard Control grant, which has assisted with the repair of many properties.

Limitations/problems encountered: Many landlords were initially unresponsive to the city's interest in paint, arguing that it was not a safety issue. Resistance dissipated as it became apparent that the City would not be deterred regarding deteriorated paint.

Magnitude of Impact/Potential Impact: Approximately 1500 rental properties are inspected each year. The majority are cited for paint violations, and the deteriorated paint is repaired.

Potential for replication: Moderate. Can be replicated wherever there is a property maintenance code that the City is willing to enforce.

Contact for Specific Information
Kathy Lamb
Senior Housing Inspector
563-589-4231
klamb@cityofdubuque.org

References for additional information
1. City of Dubuque website—Housing section
   www.cityofdubuque.org

ILLUSTRATION #2 OF STRATEGY IN PRACTICE

An ordinance passed in 2002 gave code inspectors the authority to pursue charges against property owners who do not treat lead-based paint hazards in their buildings. The City of Kankakee's Community Development Agency's Lead Poisoning Prevention Program (LPPP) trained code inspectors to visually assess and identify lead hazards. When code inspectors discover an existing or potential lead hazard, they can refer the property owner to the LPPP. Through its HUD Healthy Homes grant, the program helps property owners make repairs before a hazard develops, as well as remediate or abate existing hazards. Property owners who do not follow up on the voluntary referral are cited.

Jurisdiction or Target Area: Kankakee, IL

Primary Actor: Kankakee Community Development Agency, Lead Poisoning Prevention Program.

Secondary Actor(s): N/A

Staffing utilized: No information provided.

Other resources utilized: No information provided.

Factors essential to implementation: A good relationship with the code enforcement division is key. Outreach to property owners through local landlord association allowed them to address concerns up front as well and educate property owners about lead hazards before inspections. HUD Healthy Homes and CDBG monies provide the funding to assist property owners in lead-safe work practices and lead hazard remediation.

Limitations/challenges/problems encountered: Occasionally a property owner doesn't recognize the seriousness of the problem, but the LPPP grants typically alleviate any objections. Nominal outreach was needed to bring the Code Enforcement Division and the Health Department together, since each agency has its own focus.

Magnitude of Impact/Potential Impact: LPPP receives an average of 20-25 referrals per month. In its first two-year grant cycle, it assisted 300 properties and will complete another 240 this cycle. As a result of interactions with code inspectors, other property owners voluntarily contact LPPP for lead hazard information and assistance. Outreach coordinators have seen a shift in community awareness also, from landlord association meetings to WIC outreach.

Potential for replication: Moderate. This strategy can be replicated wherever there is a property maintenance code that the city is willing to enforce.

Contacts for Specific Information

Jenny Rodriguez
Community Coordinator
815-933-0488
cdajlr@keynet.net

Steve Lanter
Lead Grant Manager
815-936-3623
cdasel@keynet.net

References for additional information
1. City of Kankakee, Municipal Code, Property Maintenance Code, Chapter 8, §8-24(c).

INFORM RENTAL PROPERTY OWNERS OF FEDERAL LEAD HAZARD DISCLOSURE REQUIREMENTS

DESCRIPTION OF THE STRATEGY

The federal lead hazard disclosure Law requires property owners to provide information on lead poisoning and known property-specific data to tenants upon lease or lease renewal. Many rental property owners are unaware of the law and/or are out of compliance. Community-based organizations (CBOs) or governmental agencies can mail boilerplate letters to rental property owners with information on federal lead hazard disclosure requirements, applicable local laws, and available resources, such as free lead-safe work practices training and lead hazard control grant funds. Agencies and organizations with access to property-specific information related to lead-based paint and hazards can send registered letters that put owners on notice about specific hazards and remind them that this information must be provided to tenants. Other ways to reach out to landlords include seminars, one-on-one meetings, and notices included in water or other bills. Sending complementary mailings to tenants, especially those in units with known lead hazards, puts increased pressure on landlords and further protects tenants by informing them of their rights and providing them with information their landlord may be withholding.

BENEFITS

Immediate/Direct Results: Providing information about landlord responsibilities under the federal lead hazard disclosure law will increase owner compliance and motivate some owners to take measures to control hazards—especially if resources are available to help them (e.g., training in lead-safe work practices and lead hazard control grants and loans).

Public Health Benefits: Tenants will receive information they need to make informed housing choices and protect their families from lead.

Other Indirect/Collateral Benefits: Reaching out to landlords will help agencies and organizations identify cooperative owners who will benefit from assistance and put them in a position to monitor unresponsive landlords. Also, demand for lead-safe work practices training and enrollment in lead hazard control programs will increase; these programs traditionally have experienced difficulties attracting owners of high-risk properties.

SCOPE OF POTENTIAL IMPACT

Statewide   Regional (e.g. multi-county)
City- or County-Wide   Neighborhood/Community

PRIMARY ACTORS

Health Department
Code or Building Inspection Agency
Housing Agency
Property Owners

KEY PARTNERS

Code Enforcement Agencies
Community-based Organizations

CRITICAL ELEMENTS

Staff requirements: 0.5 – 1.25 FTEs for mailings and providing follow-up assistance, depending on ease of access to data and the amount of follow-up assistance provided.

Other resource requirements: Access to a variety of databases and types of information to identify owners of pre-1978 housing in high-risk communities and properties with known lead hazards, such as: tax assessor records, EBL data, housing code violations, GIS data, and inspection and risk assessment results.

Institutional capacity required: Ability to provide follow-up assistance to landlords and monitor lead hazard control activities.

Cost considerations: Mailings are a relatively low-cost way to reach out to landlords. However, there must be time and resources allocated to provide follow-up assistance and a plan for follow-up contact with unresponsive owners.

Timing issues: The entire process, from the research through the mailing stage, can be implemented in less than six months. Follow-up could take a year or more.

Feasibility of Implementation: High. Fairly easy to implement by any jurisdiction.

POTENTIAL OBSTACLES/BARRIERS

Identifying and locating the owner of high-risk rental properties is often difficult. Identifying properties with known lead hazards is challenging, particularly for CBOs.

ADDITIONAL RESOURCES

1. Model "Boilerplate" Letter
   www.afhh.org/res/res_pubs/disclosure_model_boilerplate_letter.doc
2. Model Registered Letter
   www.afhh.org/res/res_pubs/disclosure_res_model_registered_letter.doc
3. Complying with the Federal Lead Hazard Disclosure Law: A Guide for Rental Property Owners and Managers
   www.afhh.org/res/res_pubs/disclosure_landlord_requirements.doc

4. Lynn Battle
   Citizens' Lead Education Poisoning Prevention
   205-780-8077
   wbattle@bellsouth.net

5. Lorisa Seibel
   Durham Affordable Housing Coalition
   919-683-1185, ext. 25
   lorisa@dahc.org

6. Tom Neltner
   Improving Kids' Environment
   317-283-5648
   neltner@ikecoalition.org

7. New Jersey Citizen Action
   732-246-4772

8. Carolyn Gillam
   Clark County Combined Health District
   937-390-5600
   cchdlead@iapdatacom.net

9. Rita Gergely
   Iowa Department of Public Health
   515-242-6340
   rgergely@health.state.ia.us

10. Joe Diorio
    Mahoning County District Board of Health
    330-270-2855, ext. 142
    jdiorio@mahoning-health.org

11. Ed Norman
    North Carolina Children's Environmental Health Branch
    919-715-3293
    Ed.Norman@ncmail.net

ILLUSTRATION #1 OF STRATEGY IN PRACTICE

In the City of Cleveland, all water bills, by law, must be sent to property owners (not tenants). With funding through a national project funded by a HUD Operation LEAP grant, the Cleveland Department of Public Health has developed a flyer on the lead hazard disclosure law to be included in water bill mailings. It is estimated that 450,000 flyers will be mailed. A website and hotline have been established to respond to owners who want assistance or need more information.

Jurisdiction or Target Area: Cleveland

Primary Actor: Cleveland Department of Public Health

Secondary Actor(s): Cleveland Fair Housing Office and Cleveland Water Authority.

Staffing utilized: Approximately 1-1.5 FTEs, including time to design and produce the flyer, set up the website and hotline, and staff the hotline. The Lead Hazard Control Program Manager developed the notice in cooperation with Cleveland Fair Housing Office.

Other resources utilized: N/A

Factors essential to implementation: Partnerships with the Cleveland Fair Housing Office and the Cleveland Water Authority.

Limitations/challenges/problems encountered: None listed.

Magnitude of Impact/Potential Impact: The owners of 450,000 properties serviced by the Cleveland Water Authority will be informed of their responsibilities under the federal lead hazard disclosure law and the Fair Housing Act. It is not possible to predict how many will take additional steps, like visit the website, call the hotline, and take steps to control lead hazards.

Potential for replication: Very high

Contact for Specific Information
Jonathon Brandt
Lead Hazard Control Program Manager
216-664-4939
jbrandt@city.cleveland.oh.us

References for additional information
N/A

ILLUSTRATION #2 OF STRATEGY IN PRACTICE

With funding from a HUD Operation LEAP grant, CCRG has developed and mailed 300 boilerplate and 213 registered letters to owners of high-risk rental properties in Hartford. 300 properties were identified through CCRG's treatment center/lead safe house, which provides services for children with EBLs of 20 μg/dl or above. An additional 200 properties were identified through CCRG's Community Environmental Health Resource Center (CEHRC) project. 100 landlords responded to the letters by calling CCRG with questions, and many requested additional information about lead-safe work practices training and funding for lead hazard control. Other owners have requested meetings to learn more about their responsibilities under disclosure and information on lead-safe work practices training and funds for hazard control. At the behest of property owners, CCRG is developing a seminar on disclosure and the state lead hazard control grant program and is working to schedule a free training in lead-safe work practices.

Jurisdiction or Target Area: Hartford, Connecticut

Primary Actor: Connecticut Citizens Research Group (CCRG)

Secondary Actor(s): N/A

Staffing utilized: 0.5-1 FTEs to research, prepare, and mail letters and provide follow-up assistance to responsive owners.

Other resources utilized: City of Hartford Assessor's Office database.

Factors essential to implementation: Resources to offer follow-up assistance to property owners.

Limitations/challenges/problems encountered: Difficulty securing EBL addresses from local health departments because of HIPAA concerns.

Magnitude of Impact/Potential Impact: It is apparent that a number of property owners will be trained in lead-safe work practices and enroll in the lead hazard control grant program as a result of this outreach effort.

Potential for replication: Very high

Contact for Specific Information
Sherrill Coleman
860-525-1834, ext. 26
scoleman@ccag.net

References for additional information
N/A

ILLUSTRATION #3 OF STRATEGY IN PRACTICE

GHC mails out "boilerplate" letters to landlords owning pre-1978 properties in high-risk areas. The letters inform owners about lead poisoning, lead hazards, and their duties under the disclosure law. The letter invites landlords to a free dinner, where they can learn more about lead issues. Representatives of the Health Department, Code Enforcement, Fair Housing, and Lead Hazard Control Program make presentations and provide handouts at these dinners, and certificates for free clearance testing are given out as door prizes.

Approximately 25% of the owners contacted via letters have attended dinners, and GHC is starting to receive responses from previously uncooperative owners.

Jurisdiction or Target Area: Greensboro, North Carolina

Primary Actor: Greensboro Housing Coalition (GHC)

Secondary Actor(s): N/A

Staffing utilized: 0.25 – 0.5 FTEs for four mailings and eight dinners, including researching and preparing the mailings and planning for and convening the dinners.

Other resources utilized: Data sources include information collected during GHC's neighborhood outreach and hazard assessment activities (as a subcontractor to CEHRC and the city's lead hazard control program), the city's housing code enforcement database, and the tax assessor's database. GHC uses a laptop and digital projector for presentations. A transitional housing program with a large community room donates space for the meetings. Food is purchased and prepared by GHC staff.

Factors essential to implementation: A key factor is good working partnerships with the range of agencies that need to communicate with landlords about their responsibilities under federal, state, and local laws, and resources available to help them make their properties lead-safe.

Limitations/challenges/problems encountered: The majority of landlords have not yet responded to the letters. Also, it has been difficult to identify and locate some owners. It is difficult to determine owners' follow up activities for two reasons: the city's lead hazard control program is overwhelmed and cannot always provide accurate and up-to-date information on the applications received; and the owners tend to not readily provide information on what, if any, steps they have taken to control lead hazards.

Magnitude of Impact/Potential Impact: Many more owners of high-risk housing are following the disclosure law. At least 25 properties have been enrolled in the city's lead hazard control grant program.

Potential for replication: Moderate

Contact for Specific Information
Beth McKee-Huger
Executive Director
336-691-9521
rachelltv@aol.com

References for additional information
N/A

ILLUSTRATION #4 OF STRATEGY IN PRACTICE

Project 504 built an extensive database of owners of pre-1950 properties in high-risk neighborhoods and is using it to mail out at least 1,000 boilerplate and 250 registered letters. Owners receiving boilerplate letters first receive a postcard to alert them to the coming letter. The postcard serves two purposes: getting the property owners' attention and culling bad addresses from the database before the more expensive letters are sent. Both the postcard and the letters refer owners to Project 504's new website designed to provide resources to property owners, www.nomorelead.org. When rental property owners contact Project 504 for more information, they are sent a letter with an accompanying stamped postcard that the owner can send directly into the county for more information on how to enroll in the lead hazard control (LHC) grant program. The county saves these cards and forwards them back to Project 504 so they can track referrals and later follow up to find out what happened with the property.

Jurisdiction or Target Area: Minneapolis, MN

Primary Actor: Project 504

Secondary Actor(s): N/A

Staffing utilized: 1-1.25 FTEs for research, setting up the database, drafting letters, preparing mailings, providing follow-up assistance to owners, and monitoring lead hazard control activities.

Other resources utilized: Data on code violations for chipping and peeling paint over the last five years were obtained through a "request for data" to the code enforcement agency. Properties with documented hazards were identified through Project 504's CEHRC project. Also, local GIS data to identify owners.

Factors essential to implementation: The website is relatively inexpensive and takes enormous pressure off Project 504 staff by minimizing the number of calls from landlords and the number of hard copies of documents sent out by mail. Having resources (e.g., lead-safe work practices training and the LHC program) to offer to property owners is key to owner responsiveness and building Project 504's credibility with this audience.

Limitations/challenges/problems encountered: Identifying properties with known hazards.

Magnitude of Impact/Potential Impact: In response to the first batch of letters that went to 257 owners, a dozen owners of multiple properties receiving these letters have contacted the county's lead hazard control program.

Potential for replication: High

Contact for Specific Information:
Greg Luce
612-521-8888
gluce@project504.org

References for additional information
N/A

PRECLUDE OWNERS FROM RENTING UNITS THAT HAVE BEEN CITED FOR HAZARDS

DESCRIPTION OF THE STRATEGY

Prohibiting owners from renting dwellings that have been cited for lead hazards provides a strong incentive for owners to address the hazards. A jurisdiction can issue an order to vacate (or even cite the unit as unfit for human occupancy) and declare those units uninhabitable. Jurisdictions that require rental licenses or certificates of occupancy can revoke them for cited units to achieve the same end. A prohibition of occupancy must be coupled with measures to protect tenants from eviction, offer relocation assistance when absolutely necessary, and safeguard against possible loss of affordable housing due to gentrification.

BENEFITS

Immediate/Direct Results: With the potential loss of rental income, property owners will be motivated to remediate hazards.

Public Health Benefits: Hazards will be removed and fewer children will be poisoned. Rental housing will meet minimum standards, resulting in healthier and safer housing.

Other Indirect/Collateral Benefits: More public awareness regarding lead hazards, lead poisoning, and lead poisoning prevention.

SCOPE OF POTENTIAL IMPACT

City- or County-Wide   Neighborhood/Community

PRIMARY ACTORS

Building or Code Inspection Agency

KEY PARTNERS

Housing Agency
Federal Agencies

CRITICAL ELEMENTS

Staff requirements: Additional staffing may be needed to process paperwork such as notices and placards, re-inspect units, and, after violations are cured, approve properties for reoccupancy.

Institutional capacity required: Local code must stipulate that a certificate of occupancy is required for all rental property and contingent on compliance with minimum property maintenance standards.

Timing issues: Officials must be realistic about the start-up time needed for initial inspections and certifications.

Feasibility of Implementation: It is helpful for the local jurisdiction to have funding for grants and low-cost loans available to help owners make repairs. Also, partnerships with community organizations to provide outreach and educational materials for property owners can help landlords come into compliance before inspections, thereby minimizing tenant displacement.

POTENTIAL OBSTACLES/BARRIERS

Without funding for grants and loans and in the absence of local community group partnerships to provide education and outreach to property owners, code enforcement officials may issue a great deal of citations initially, which may increase tensions with property owners. Also, whatever database is used to identify rental units must be current in order to reach as many properties as possible.

ADDITIONAL RESOURCES

1. ICC International Property Code §301.1 and §304.3

ILLUSTRATION OF STRATEGY IN PRACTICE

As of January 2004, Greensboro requires all residential property owners to acquire and maintain a valid Rental Unit Certificate of Occupancy (CO) before the property can be rented or leased. Units that meet the International Property Maintenance Code minimum standards on the first inspection (or re-inspection within 45 days) get a free five-year CO. Units that do not meet the standards within 45 days must be vacated until the unit is brought into compliance; at this point, owners must pay $250 for the CO. With additional complaints, the costs rise. Once the unit has a CO, if a complaint inspection results in a violation, the unit must be vacated. Owners must then repair within 45 days and pay $500 to restore the CO. The next verified complaint also results in a revoked CO and a vacated unit, but restoring the CO will cost $500 plus $25 for each day that the unit is out of compliance.

The IPMC lists peeling and deteriorating paint as a violation. When an inspector cites a property for paint violations, the owner is referred to the housing and community development program to apply for a lead hazard control grant. A local non-profit, the Greensboro Housing Coalition (GHC), also provides outreach to landlords to educate them about minimum standards and help them find solutions for rental property problems. GHC is also prepared to assist displaced tenants.

Jurisdiction or Target Area: Greensboro, NC

Primary Actor: Greensboro, NC, Engineering & Inspections Department, Local Ordinance Enforcement (LOE) program

Secondary Actor(s): N/A

Staffing utilized: Greensboro implemented the RUCO program with existing staff, but added one full-time program assistant; three part-time inspectors were also brought on to take over other department projects. Six full-time inspectors average between eight and 10 inspections per day; they expect to inspect the city's 45,000 rental units by 2009.

Other resources utilized: The Greensboro code enforcement program used this opportunity to revamp software and purchase new notepad computers for mobile operations.

Factors essential to implementation: A requirement that all rental property receive a certificate of occupancy that is dependent on property maintenance code compliance.

Limitations/challenges/problems encountered: Greensboro's existing rental unit database was not current, so they had to develop a new database. The number of requests by property owners for inspections, in lieu of waiting until the inspectors reach that area of the city, exceeded the city's expectations.

Magnitude of Impact/Potential: Greensboro implemented RUCO in January 2004, so the actual impact cannot yet be measured. However, prior to RUCO, there were no negative consequences for landlords who do not respond promptly to repair orders. With a real tracking system in place with very clear consequences (i.e. loss of rental income), local code enforcers believe there will be a dramatic and permanent change in Greensboro rental housing.

Potential for replication: Once the ordinance was passed, there were no significant additional burdens to overcome, making this a simple yet effective strategy to replicate.

Contact for Specific Information

Dan Reynolds
Inspections Division Manager
336-412-6216
dan.reynolds@greensboro-nc.gov

Beth McKee-Huger
Greensboro Housing Coalition
336-691-9521
RachellTv@aol.com

References for additional information

1. Greensboro, NC, Code of Ordinances §11-40 (1961) (effective Jan. 1, 2004)

REPORT PROBLEM RENTAL PROPERTY OWNERS TO HUD AND EPA FOR DISCLOSURE ENFORCEMENT

DESCRIPTION OF THE STRATEGY

Federal law requires owners of most pre-1978 rental properties to disclose information about lead hazards to tenants at the time of lease or lease renewal. The law provides significant penalties for violations and authorizes enforcement by HUD, EPA, and DOJ. Using "results-oriented" enforcement, federal agencies have investigated cases referred by local agencies and others and generated $14,000,000 in lead safety investments by landlords in 150,000 housing units. Health departments and community-based organizations can facilitate enforcement locally by identifying and reporting owners of poorly maintained buildings who fail to comply with disclosure requirements to EPA, HUD, or US attorneys. Health departments can strengthen federal enforcement by providing information on documented poisonings and lead hazards in non-compliant properties.

BENEFITS

Immediate/Direct Results: Landlords who have violated the federal lead hazard disclosure law are encouraged to evaluate, control, and prevent lead hazards in multiple units in exchange for reduced fines.

Public Health Benefits: Tenants living in units where hazards have been controlled or prevented are less likely to be exposed to lead hazards. Future tenants will receive information they need to make informed housing choices and protect their families from lead hazards. Owners forced to follow the disclosure law will be motivated to address lead hazards to avoid having to disclose them.

Other Indirect/Collateral Benefits: This is a good way to target problem landlords, particularly owners of properties responsible for repeat poisonings. If federal agencies pursue results-oriented enforcement, working with federal authorities in bringing enforcement actions against property owners may persuade landlords to address lead hazards in all units they own or manage as well as yield funding for education, outreach, screening, and other prevention activities. Through Community Health Improvement Projects (CHIPs) and Supplemental Environmental Projects (SEPs), a few large and well-publicized enforcement cases will also get the attention of other property owners and hopefully motivate them to comply with the disclosure law and address lead hazards in their properties.

SCOPE OF POTENTIAL IMPACT

Statewide

City- or County-Wide

Regional (e.g. multi-county)

Neighborhood/Community

PRIMARY ACTORS

Health Department

Community-based Organizations

KEY PARTNERS

Code or Building Inspection Agency

Property Taxation Agency

Attorney General

HUD, DOJ, and/or EPA

Tenants

CRITICAL ELEMENTS

Staff requirements: Number of FTEs can vary greatly, depending on the level of involvement of the agency reporting violations. Simply reporting violations identified in the course of regular activities entails very little extra work. Systematically providing information on EBLs, the presence of lead hazards, code violations, and documentation of disclosure violations; profiling owners; intervening in the enforcement action; and influencing settlements to ensure they include projects needed by the affected community may require 1-2 FTEs per year over two or more years.

Other resource requirements: N/A

Institutional capacity required: Address-specific information about lead hazards is necessary. Access to EBL data, tax assessor's records, and data on housing code and other violations is helpful. Local or state lead laws are not required for the implementation of this strategy.

Cost considerations: This is a very cost-effective strategy—a relatively small investment of time and resources can reap tens of thousands of dollars in property owner investments in lead safety and other prevention projects. There is no evidence that results-oriented enforcement of the disclosure law has adversely affected housing affordability.

Timing issues: Typically, it can take more than one year for federal agencies to complete enforcement action, from the investigation through the settlement stage; some cases may take even longer. It can take another two or more years for defendants to complete the work agreed to in the settlements.

Feasibility of Implementation: Very high. This is an easy strategy for local and state entities to implement, because federal agencies conduct the investigation and enforcement work once cases are referred.

POTENTIAL OBSTACLES/BARRIERS

Some tenants may be reluctant to report non-compliance or provide documentation for fear of landlord retaliation. It is important to communicate these fears when reporting cases for enforcement to federal agencies so that steps can be taken to protect tenants and safeguard their rights.

Also, follow-up monitoring is needed to ensure that landlords implement settlement agreements properly. Federal agencies have the ability to collect penalties if agreements are not honored.

ADDITIONAL RESOURCES

1. Marcheta Gillam
    Legal Aid Society of Cincinnati
    513-241-9400
    mgillam@lascinti.org

2. Lorisa Seibel
    Durham Affordable Housing Coalition
    919-683-1185, ext. 25
    lorisa@dahc.org

3. Beth McKee-Huger
    Greensboro Housing Coalition
    336-691-9046
    rachelltv@aol.com

4. Tom Neltner
    Improving Kids' Environment
    317-283-6111
    neltner@ikecoalition.org

5. Linda Kite
    Healthy Homes Collaborative
    213-386-4901, ext. 107
    lkite@psr.org

6. Joe Diorio
    Mahoning County District Board of Health
    330-270-2855, ext. 142
    jdiorio@mahoning-health.org

7. New Jersey Citizen Action
    732-246-4772

8. Ed Norman
    North Carolina Children's Environmental Health Branch
    919-715-3293
    Ed.Norman@ncmail.net

9. Strategies for Making the Most of the Federal Lead Hazard Disclosure Law
    www.afhh.org/res/res_pubs/disclosure_strategies_paper.pdf

10. Guide to Identifying and Documenting Disclosure Law Violations
    www.afhh.org/res/res_pubs/disclosure_documenting_violations_guide.pdf

11. Innovative SEPs and CHIPs for Inclusion in Lead Hazard Disclosure Settlements
    www.afhh.org/res/res_pubs/disclosure_Innovative_SEPs_and_CHIPs.pdf

---

ILLUSTRATION #1 OF STRATEGY IN PRACTICE

CDPH, HUD, DOJ, EPA Region 5, and the Illinois Department of Public Health entered into discussions regarding disclosure enforcement. CDPH identified owners and management companies of properties with large numbers of EBL children and frequent and repeat violations of Chicago's municipal code requirement that all properties be maintained in a lead-safe manner. HUD and EPA investigated whether disclosure had occurred in these properties. Where disclosure violations were found, CDPH performed additional inspections, which added the threat of municipal actions to the negotiations over the federal violations. These activities resulted in four settlements. CDPH has begun the process again with new property management companies/owners in violation of local laws.

Jurisdiction or Target Area: Chicago

Primary Actor: Chicago Department of Public Health (CDPH)

Secondary Actor(s): US Environmental Protection Agency, US Department of Housing and Urban Development, US Department of Justice

Staffing utilized: Approximately 0.75 FTEs per year over 2 years, including an epidemiologist, clerks, the director of the program, attorneys, and inspectors.

Other resources utilized: Tax assessor's database.

Factors essential to implementation: The key components are a clean database of EBLs and local law violations, a good working relationship with federal enforcement officials, and a strong local lead law.

Limitations/challenges/problems encountered: HUD typically takes the lead in monitoring implementation of the agreements but does not have the resources to monitor all cases nationally; CDPH is involved, but does not have dedicated funding for this activity.

Magnitude of Impact/Potential Impact: The four companies agreed to conduct lead hazard control in a total of 8,642 units at an estimated cost of $6 million. To date, 477 units have been made lead safe and more than $750,000 has been spent on testing and abatement. In addition, the settlements included $77,000 for blood lead screening and $100,000 for abatement of 10 housing units owned by low-income property owners.

Potential for replication: Low. Unless there is a strong local law and resources to proactively inspect properties, it would be difficult for health departments to fully replicate the Chicago experience—but many elements are worth replicating.

Contacts for Specific Information

Anne Evens
Director, CLPPP
312-746-7820
Evens_Anne@cdph.org

Tara Jordan
National Center for Healthy Housing
410-992-0712
tara.jordan@centerforhealthyhousing.org

References for additional information
N/A

ILLUSTRATION #2 OF STRATEGY IN PRACTICE

Through health department data, the tax assessor's database, and a number of other data sources, Brown University students working for CLAP were able to determine that of 887 properties owned by 204 owners had poisoned 2,644 children. CLAP profiled these owners, documented disclosure violations in their properties, and provided this information to the Attorney General's office, which in turn prioritized the cases and forwarded them to EPA Region 1. CLAP continues to document and report disclosure violations as tenants provide tips.

Jurisdiction or Target Area: Rhode Island

Primary Actor: Childhood Lead Action Project (CLAP)

Secondary Actor(s): EPA Region 1

Staffing utilized: 1 to 1.5 FTEs per year, over four years.

Other resources utilized: Brown University students did much of the initial research. Through a contract between Brown University and the Rhode Island Department of Health, the students had access to health department EBL data. The information they compiled was sent directly to the federal agencies.

Factors essential to implementation: Important components are a good working relationship with the AG's Office, as well as networking and building relationships with various agencies to gain access to records.

Limitations/challenges/problems encountered: EPA Region 1 is now poised to act on the cases referred by CLAP—two years after CLAP supplied the documentation.

Magnitude of Impact/Potential Impact: So far, one case has been prosecuted, resulting in abatement of 12 units plus the contribution of $3,000 for community-based organizations working on lead poisoning prevention. In addition, the owner was fined $16,000 and was required to make five presentations about lead-based paint hazards: three to tenants and two to landlords.

Potential for Replication: Very high. Any state or local health departments could easily replicate CLAP's strategy since they have ready access to EBL data.

Contact for Specific Information

Liz Colon
Organizing Director
401-785-1310
organizingdirector@leadsafekids.org

References for additional information

N/A

REQUIRE AGENCIES TO DISSEMINATE LEAD POISONING PREVENTION INFORMATION

DESCRIPTION OF THE STRATEGY

Requiring governmental agencies that have regular contact with homeowners, landlords, tenants, and parents to disseminate lead poisoning prevention information to their constituents is an effective way to advance primary prevention. Agencies can enclose information on lead poisoning prevention when they mail items such as property tax statements and water and utility bills or when they provide such documents as birth certificates and building permits. This is an effective, low-cost method that can use existing systems and leverage limited funding while distributing lead poisoning prevention information to thousands of people.

BENEFITS

Immediate/Direct Results: Lead poisoning prevention information disseminated by public agencies instantly reaches thousands of people who receive property tax bills and pay water and other utility bills.

Public Health Benefits: Especially as tied to building permits, this strategy can alert homeowners and rental property owners about the hazards that could be created by disturbing or removing lead-based paint, as well as educate these groups about lead-safe work practices; both are measures that can protect public health. This strategy can also alert parents to potential lead hazards and what steps are needed to protect their children from lead hazards.

Other Indirect/Collateral Benefits: This effort can raise awareness about the extent of lead hazards in a community and potentially generate interest in lead hazard control strategies.

SCOPE OF POTENTIAL IMPACT

Statewide   City- or County-Wide

Neighborhood/Community

PRIMARY ACTORS

Health Department

Code or Building Inspection Agency

Housing Agency

Property Taxation Agency

Medicaid Agency

Public Water Utility

School District

Public Libraries

KEY PARTNERS

Community-based Organizations

Property Owners

Tenants

Utilities

CRITICAL ELEMENTS

Staff requirements: No new staff time should be required; a small percentage of an FTE would be needed to produce and distribute the information materials to the participating agencies.

Other resource requirements: The information materials to be enclosed with mailings or document distribution.

Institutional capacity required: This strategy may require statutory or code authority. It also requires a knowledgeable staff member to compile the information materials and to ensure that all agencies have all required materials for dissemination.

Cost considerations: The cost of producing the materials: writing, editing, graphics, reproduction, and the incremental cost of collating the document(s) into the other material the disseminating agency was already distributing.

Timing issues: Once underlying statutory or code authority is in place, implementation of this strategy should be very quick.

Feasibility of Implementation: This strategy should be very easy to implement at any level.

POTENTIAL OBSTACLES/BARRIERS

A potential challenge is whether property owners and others who receive the information with water or utility bills pay attention to the material they receive.

ADDITIONAL RESOURCES

N/A

ILLUSTRATION OF STRATEGY IN PRACTICE

As part of a larger childhood lead poisoning prevention program passed in 1991, the City and County of San Francisco directed the Department of Public Health and its CLPP to put together a collection of information materials that were then disseminated to various audiences by a number of different city and county agencies. This dissemination was required by law (city health code) and involved the public health department, the Tax Collector, the city's water utility, the San Francisco Unified School district, and others.

Two very successful portions of this policy expired in 2003. The first was a requirement to include lead hazard notices in each county tax bill. These notices included an official lead hazard Informational Bulletin, as well as a Pre-1978 Hazard Notice, both prepared by the Department of Public Health. The second portion required that all rental property owners with a unit or units constructed before 1978 distribute the official Hazard Notice to all tenants; the property owners had to retain affidavits as proof of distribution.

Other requirements still in effect include the following: the birth records office must provide bilingual lead poisoning prevention information with every birth certificate issued; the San Francisco Unified School District, the departments of Social Services and Recreation & Parks, Head Start providers, and libraries disseminate the Informational Bulletin; and city-funded child care and health care facilities are required to distribute information on lead poisoning prevention.

Jurisdiction or Target Area: City and County of San Francisco

Primary Actor: San Francisco Dept. of Public Health, San Francisco Childhood Lead Prevention Program (CLPP)

Secondary Actors: City and County Tax Collector, Public Utilities Commission, School District, Birth Records office, Departments of Social Services, Department of Recreation and Parks, Head Start providers, Public Library

Staffing utilized: All materials were produced in-house by the Department of Public Health and CLPP utilizing existing staff members.

Factors essential to implementation: The main factor essential to the implementation of this strategy was the cooperation demonstrated by all departments involved in the information dissemination process.

Limitations/challenges/problems: None

Magnitude of Impact/Potential Impact: This strategy has impacted thousands of families each year since its implementation. Staff at the CLPP estimate that when all portions of the strategy were in effect, lead poisoning prevention information was reaching between 70,000 and 100,000 households every year.

Potential for replication: The San Francisco CLPP strongly recommends this strategy to other local governments as an easy-to-implement, effective way to increase knowledge of childhood lead poisoning prevention.

Contact for Specific Information

Karen Cohen
Director
San Francisco Childhood Lead Prevention Program
415-554-8930

References for additional information

1. San Francisco Health Code, Article 26, Secs. 1611, 1613-1616
2. San Francisco Childhood Lead Prevention Program
   www.dph.sf.ca.us/cehp/Lead/lead.htm

REQUIRE AN INSPECTION FOR LEAD-BASED PAINT HAZARDS AT TENANT TURNOVER

DESCRIPTION OF THE STRATEGY

Tenant turnover presents an excellent opportunity for deteriorated paint and other potential lead hazards to be identified and corrected because the safety and convenience of occupants are not an issue in a vacant unit. Rental property owners can be required to assess and control any lead hazards after the departing tenant leaves but before the new tenant occupies the unit.

BENEFITS

Immediate/Direct Results: Regular maintenance to correct or prevent lead-based paint hazards reduces the risk of child exposure to lead.

Public Health Benefits: Triggering corrective action by landlords at the time of vacancy institutionalizes lead safety and primary prevention.

Other Indirect/Collateral Benefits: The overall quality of rental housing is improved. Property owners that perform turnover treatments may avoid the high cost of lead abatement that may be required if a child is poisoned and benefit from increased liability protection and lower insurance premiums.

SCOPE OF POTENTIAL IMPACT

Statewide   City- or County-wide

PRIMARY ACTORS

Inspection, Code, or Building Agency
Property Owners

KEY PARTNERS

Tenants

CRITICAL ELEMENTS

Staff requirements: The number of staff needed depends on the size of the jurisdiction and number of rental units.

Other resource requirements: A database of rental housing must exist or be created. Some enforcement presence is needed to monitor and enforce compliance.

Institutional capacity required: Statute, ordinance, or code that requires assessment and control at the time of or prior to tenant turnover; statutory authority to enforce such requirements; and enough code inspectors to implement it.

Cost considerations: Costs associated with creating and maintaining a rental property database; salary and other costs related to monitoring and enforcement.

Feasibility of Implementation: Variable. For jurisdictions with an existing rental property database and an active code enforcement program, this strategy has the potential to generate profound change with little cost. Jurisdictions with weak code enforcement programs will find this strategy difficult to implement.

POTENTIAL OBSTACLES/BARRIERS

Since it is impossible for code inspectors to know when rental property is turning over, this strategy's success depends on substantial voluntary property owner compliance as well as an educated renter population. Also, turnover treatment may be difficult in tight rental markets where new tenants need to occupy units quickly – such as "on the first of the month" because the leases on their previous homes expired the day before.

ADDITIONAL RESOURCES

1. R.I. Gen. Laws §42-128.1-4(5)

ILLUSTRATION OF STRATEGY IN PRACTICE

As part of statutorily mandated Essential Maintenance Practices (EMPs), Vermont law requires owners of pre-1978 rental housing to perform visual, on-site inspections on each rental unit at tenant turnover. The EMPs require, among other things, the inspection of paint condition, including interior and exterior surfaces and fixtures, and the completion of any needed repair. The essential maintenance work must be completed according to safe work practices. Owners must sign a notarized affidavit stating that EMPs have been completed and file it with their insurance carrier and the Vermont Department of Health. In Burlington, VT (the only jurisdiction currently enforcing this law), code enforcement officers conduct workshops to educate landlords about the requirements and how to meet them. The training addresses the property owners' business sense and self-interest by emphasizing that compliance with the regular property maintenance requirements placates insurance companies, protects the property, and shields property owners from liability. Burlington also does periodic mailings with detailed materials on lead paint regulations and includes the Department of Health form.

Jurisdiction or Target Area: Vermont

Primary Actor: Department of Health; Code Enforcement Office

Secondary Actor(s): N/A

Staffing utilized: Burlington did not require additional staffing.

Other resources utilized: N/A

Factors essential to implementation: An existing database of rental property or the means to create one; educational outreach materials for property owners; and sufficient staffing to conduct outreach to property owners and property maintenance companies, monitor for compliance, and enforcement

Limitations/challenges/problems encountered: Local jurisdictions other than Burlington do not have code enforcement programs or rental property databases in place and have been unable to enforce the law thus far. Also, the insurance industry's failure to support the law (although its part was voluntary) precludes the EMPs' proponents envisioned incentive for property owners to conduct an inspection and obtain a notarized affidavit.

Magnitude of Impact/Potential Impact: There is potential for tremendous impact—regular property maintenance and yearly inspections may be the best method of primary prevention. Burlington Code Enforcement finds that most property owners already inspect at tenant turnover, so educating them about the lead paint requirements is often all that is necessary for compliance.

Potential for replication: High in a location with a rental property database and sufficient staffing to do landlord outreach and monitoring.

Contacts for Specific Information

Amy Sayre
Director, Childhood Lead Poisoning Prevention Program
802-863-7388
asayre@vdh.state.vt.us

Kathleen Butler
Assistant Director, Burlington Code Enforcement Office
802-865-7510
kbutler@ci.burlington.vt.us

References for additional information

1. Vt. Stat. Ann. tit. 18, § 1759(a)

REQUIRE RENTAL PROPERTY REGISTRATION/LICENSING

DESCRIPTION OF THE STRATEGY

Universal registration or licensing of multi-unit residential buildings with state or local code enforcement authorities helps to ensure that minimum property maintenance standards are met by landlords, particularly absentee landlords. As part of the registration/licensing obligation, owners can be required to provide contact information for themselves, as well as any agents managing the property, and to designate an agent to receive legal notices in the locality where the property is situated.

BENEFITS

Immediate/Direct Results: Rental registration and licensing programs ensure that persons with responsibility and authority to maintain buildings can be readily located and served with legal notices. Successful delivery of such notices ensures that non-compliant property owners have received official notification of a code violation. This expedites compliance or enforcement action to achieve compliance with applicable housing quality and maintenance standards. Tenants also benefit from being able to readily locate those responsible for maintaining their homes to inform them about potential housing-related health hazards such as peeling paint or leaks.

Public Health Benefits: Prompt and consistent enforcement of housing codes improves the likelihood of effective maintenance of rental housing, reducing the risk of lead hazards.

Other Indirect/Collateral Benefits: Other systems, such as CLPP programs, housing authorities, and public safety agencies, can use address-based data about rental housing that identifies property owners to fulfill their missions.

SCOPE OF POTENTIAL IMPACT

Statewide   City- or County-Wide

PRIMARY ACTORS

Code or Building Inspection Agency

KEY PARTNERS

Property Taxation Agency
Local Prosecutors
Property Owners
Tenants

CRITICAL ELEMENTS

Staff requirements: Staff requirements will vary depending on whether the program is adopted at a state or local level. Once a system is in place, nominal staff is required to update records and enforce orders.

Other resource requirements: Computerized information system and methods for disseminating, retrieving, and reviewing registrations.

Institutional capacity required: Statutory authority is required in order to compel property owners to register their properties. Staff training requirements are minimal.

Cost considerations: Rental registration programs are not costly. These programs can be supported by a registration fee to minimize the impact on the code enforcement program's resources and can generate income to support pro-active inspections or enforcement.

Timing issues: An initial phase-in period will be necessary, with a deadline after which owners who have not registered their properties are considered in violation of the requirements. Re-registration should be required at minimum when properties change ownership or an owner's or agent's contact information changes.

Feasibility of Implementation: Moderate. These programs can be easily implemented once statutory authority is in place. The key to their effectiveness is adequate staffing in health and/or code inspection agencies to ensure enforcement.

POTENTIAL OBSTACLES/BARRIERS

Rental registration and licensing programs are in place in a number of jurisdictions. However, in order to be effective, they must be coupled with effective enforcement and meaningful consequences for non-compliance. In New Jersey, for example, many courts will not allow an eviction case to proceed if the property is not registered. In addition, the state can file a docketed judgment for $200 per building if an owner fails to register a property.

ADDITIONAL RESOURCES

1. William "Dan" Reynolds, Code Enforcement Manager, City of Greensboro, dan.reynolds@ci.greensboro.nc.us, phone: 336-451-1054, and Beth McKee-Huger, Greensboro Housing Coalition, rachelltv@aol.com, phone: 336-691-9521 (for information on Greensboro North Carolina's recently enacted Rental Unit Certificate of Occupancy program).

ILLUSTRATION OF STRATEGY IN PRACTICE

Owners of buildings containing three or more rental units must submit a certificate of registration to BHI as well as a $10 fee per building. Owners must provide personal contact information and designate an agent, residing in the county where the property is located, who is authorized to accept notices from tenants and to receive service of process. Corporate owners must be registered to do business in New Jersey and must identify the corporation's registered agent and corporate officers. If the property is owned by a partnership, the names of all general partners must be disclosed. Mortgage holders also must be identified. Owners must provide the name and address of any managing agent, superintendent, janitor, or other person responsible for the maintenance of the property and must designate someone who can authorize expenditures for emergency repairs. New owners are required to submit a registration form within 20 days of a acquiring a property.

Jurisdiction or Target Area: New Jersey

Primary Actor: Bureau of Housing Inspection (BHI), which is part of the Division of Codes and Standards in New Jersey's Department of Community Affairs (DCA).

Secondary Actor(s): N/A

Staffing utilized: 1-2 FTE is required to update records and enforce orders.

Other resources utilized: A computer database, registration forms, and orders.

Factors essential to implementation: Strong enforcement provisions are essential to the effectiveness of the program. If an owner fails to register a property, DCA notifies the owner of the violation and orders him to register within 30 days. If the owner still neglects to comply, the Department imposes a penalty of $200 per violation and certifies the debt to the superior court. The clerk of the court immediately dockets a judgment against the owner. Implementation is also enhanced by tying rental registration requirements to the state's construction code: owners may not obtain a certificate of occupancy for newly constructed rental housing without first procuring a certificate of registration. Finally, owners may not evict tenants from buildings that are not registered.

Limitations/challenges/problems encountered: None

Magnitude of Impact/Potential Impact: All rental housing located in buildings with three or more units is subject to rental registration.

Potential for replication: Moderate

Contact for Specific Information
Amy Fenwick Frank
Section Chief, NJ DCA, Division of Codes and Standards
609-292-7899
afrank@dca.state.nj.us

References for additional information
1. New Jersey Hotel and Multiple Dwelling Law, N.J.S.A. 55:13A-1 *et seq.*
2. Alliance For Healthy Homes (formerly The Alliance To End Childhood Lead Poisoning), "Holding Property Owners Accountable: New Jersey Multiple Dwelling Registration And Inspection Program," *Innovative Strategies For Addressing Lead Hazards In Distressed And Marginal Housing: A Collection Of Best Practices*
   www.afhh.org/res/res_pubs/bp.doc.

UTILIZE EARLY WARNING SYSTEMS FOR DETERIORATING PROPERTIES

DESCRIPTION OF THE STRATEGY

An easy-to-use online tool that integrates public data about deteriorating and potentially deteriorating properties is an innovative means of leveraging code enforcement and targeting high-risk housing. Such a web site provides a searchable database of information that enables the identification of properties in danger of decline, such as code complaints, contract nuisance abatements (city-sponsored repairs to address public safety hazards), tax delinquencies, and liens for unpaid utility bills. City agencies, county agencies, and community groups can use search results to identify properties in trouble; acquire properties headed for abandonment before they deteriorate; determine if landlords are complying with obligations; and learn about the overall condition of various neighborhoods.

BENEFITS

Immediate/Direct Results: Coordinating underutilized public information delivers a comprehensive picture of what actually is happening in a particular block or neighborhood. Using a system that identifies properties likely to decline, public agencies can notify property owners about potential lead problems and require or encourage that they make repairs before problems become serious hazards and children are poisoned.

Public Health Benefits: Such a system has multiple applied uses that can prevent childhood lead poisoning: community development corporations and other groups can identify property owners in trouble and offer proactive services or acquire properties before they deteriorate; residents can determine whether their landlords are complying with their obligations and learn about patterns in their neighborhoods; and code enforcement agencies can use the information to target troubled neighborhoods, problem owners, high-risk properties and neighborhoods in decline.

Other Indirect/Collateral Benefits: Comprehensive, integrated public information—including mapping capability for visual representation of the data—provides powerful data that can be used to advance policy change. Free training and public access to the collected information bridges the digital divide and encourages the development of technical and community-organizing skills among community residents.

SCOPE OF POTENTIAL IMPACT

City- or County-Wide   Neighborhood/Community

PRIMARY ACTORS

Community-based Organizations

KEY PARTNERS*

Health Department
Code or Building Inspection Agency
Housing Agency
Property Taxation Agency
Local Prosecutors
Child Welfare Agencies
Tenants
Physicians
Parents

* Various local government agencies and utilities provide the necessary neighborhood data for other government agencies, community residents, and advocates to utilize.

CRITICAL ELEMENTS

Staff requirements: Staff are needed initially to develop the interface between multiple data sources and provide training and outreach to engage potential users. Continuing staff capacity is needed to update and maintain the information system.

Other resource requirements: The managing entity requires website management and development capabilities, computers for staff use, and a system for managing the data supplied by government agencies and other entities.

Institutional capacity required: Authority to share data is needed.

Cost considerations: Costs will vary considerably depending on whether an existing information system can be expanded to manage the co-location of multiple data sets or an entirely new system is needed to receive available data sets, and if any key sources lack automated capacity or compatible data programs. A simple system may cost between $50,000 and $100,000

Timing issues: Between 6 and 18 months is required for planning and initial implementation.

Feasibility of Implementation: Variable. This strategy could be successfully replicated by jurisdictions that have relevant data in electronic files. There must be an interested party willing and authorized to tackle the integration and centralization of the data.

POTENTIAL OBSTACLES/BARRIERS

Ambivalence and/or outright resistance from city and county agencies may be encountered. The resistance may stem from turf-protection issues, perceived additional workload, and/or reluctance to make certain information publicly accessible. Another key consideration is ensuring that the central organizing entity has the necessary capacity, knowledge, authority, and credibility to be able to engage all of the necessary players and sustain the project once in place.

ADDITIONAL RESOURCES

N/A

ILLUSTRATION OF STRATEGY IN PRACTICE

Neighborhood Knowledge Los Angeles (NKLA) is dedicated to preventing Los Angeles housing and neighborhood conditions from deteriorating. It provides a searchable, online tool, highlighted on its website, that tracks multiple data sets (including code complaints, building permits, contract nuisance abatements, tax delinquencies, and utility liens) gathered from city agencies. Tenants, community advocacy groups, and others may search the site (in English or Spanish) by zip code, census tract, council district, or address, or by specific user-selected criteria, such as properties with pending code complaint cases. Any of the site's data sets may be viewed area-wide on easy-to-read maps. This mapping function allows users to spot patterns of tax delinquencies, code complaints, or other problems indicating pockets of potential neighborhood decay. Such comprehensive and illustrative information helps neighborhood residents, community organizations, and policymakers mobilize support for community improvement.

Jurisdiction or Target Area: Los Angeles, CA

Primary Actor: Neighborhood Knowledge Los Angeles

Secondary Actor(s): N/A

Staffing utilized: NKLA had three full-time staff working on the project initially—two on training and outreach, and one dedicated to updating and maintaining the information system.

Other resources utilized: NKLA used a computer lab or local community technology center to train users at the neighborhood level.

Factors essential to implementation: The project's association with UCLA helped considerably as NKLA sought out relationships with local government agencies that possessed the needed data sets. These relationships were crucial to the project's implementation and success. NKLA has received funding from city and federal governmental authorities as well as private foundations and corporations.

Limitations/challenges/problems encountered: Initially, most of the needed data sets were spread throughout the City of Los Angeles on individual computers or inaccessible mainframe systems. Convincing the individuals involved to share the data was challenging. Staying competent in an ever-changing technology is an ongoing challenge.

Magnitude of Impact/Potential Impact: With the various data sets integrated, the scope of property deterioration was documented clearly, and city staff, politicians, and advocates were better able to grasp the need for regularized code inspection. In Oct. 2000, NKLA received about 250,000 hits each month, with approximately 100 different individual users on the site each day.

Potential for replication: Moderate. The information central to this strategy already exists in various government agencies, which makes this a promising strategy for replication. NKLA contains "A Political and Technical How-To Kit" for those seeking to replicate the site in other locales. The kit offers advice on overcoming the political as well as technical challenges confronted by the site's creators.

Contact for Specific Information

Charanjeet Singh
310-825-8886
charan@ucla.edu

References for additional information

1. Neighborhood Knowledge Los Angeles
   http://nkla.ucla.edu

APPENDICES

APPENDIX A—Template

APPENDIX B—Agencies and Organizations Included in Illustrations

APPENDIX C—Locations of Illustrations

APPENDIX D—Acronym Index

APPENDIX E—Glossary of Terms

APPENDIX A
TEMPLATE

TITLE

DESCRIPTION OF THE STRATEGY
Summary

BENEFITS
- o **Immediate/Direct Results**
- o **Public Health Benefits**
- o **Other Indirect/Collateral Benefits**

SCOPE OF POTENTIAL IMPACT
    Statewide
    Regional (e.g. multi-county)
    City- or County-Wide
    Neighborhood/Community
    Specific (Targeted) Population

PRIMARY ACTORS AND KEY PARTNERS - *Who must be at the table (or in the field)?*
    Health Department
    Inspection, Code, or Building Agency
    Housing/Community Development Agency
    Property Taxation Agency
    Human Services/Welfare/Medicaid Agency
    City/County Solicitors, Prosecutors, Judges
    Other Agencies (e.g. Water Bureau, EMT, Fire, Police, School District, Child Welfare)
    Federal Agencies
    Community-based Organizations
    Property Owners
    Tenants
    Laborers (e.g. Contractors, Day Workers, Painters)
    Retail Stores, Suppliers, Manufacturers
    Service Providers (e.g. physicians, day care providers, hospitals, utility companies)
    General Public and Consumers (e.g. parents, homebuyers, volunteers, etc.)

CRITICAL ELEMENTS
- o **Staff requirements:** *Number of FTEs*
- o **Other resource requirements:** *Equipment, Data, etc.*
- o **Institutional capacity required:** *Statutory Authority, Training, Accreditation, etc.*
- o **Cost considerations:** *Cost-effectiveness*
- o **Timing issues:** *Timeline to Implement; Duration; Seasonal or Cyclical Factors, etc.*
- o **Feasibility of Implementation**

POTENTIAL OBSTACLES/BARRIERS *that might prohibit or limit the realization of this strategy*

ADDITIONAL RESOURCES

ILLUSTRATION OF STRATEGY IN PRACTICE

Scope and particulars of the strategy: *applicability; what/where/who/when; essential regulations, statutes, or other policies; dedicated funding or budget authority*

Jurisdiction or Target Area
Agency/Organization Name of Primary Actor
Agency/Organization Name of Secondary Actor(s)
Staffing utilized: *Number of FTE staff, needed credentials*
Other resources utilized: *Equipment, data, etc.*
Factors essential to implementation *(e.g. partnerships, policies)*
Limitations/challenges/problems encountered
Magnitude of actual impact: *number of families/homes benefiting; relative to need or eligible universe; total and unit-level $*
Potential for replication *(optional if relevant content covered above)*

Contacts for Specific Information
                    Contact # 1   *Contact #2 (if there is one)*
Name
Title
Telephone
Email

References for additional information *(citations of related regulations, statutes, codes; web site; documents, etc.)*

APPENDIX B
AGENCIES AND ORGANIZATIONS INCLUDED IN ILLUSTRATIONS

Agency or Organization Partner	Web Link
State and Local Government Agencies and Programs	
Alameda County (CA) CLPPP	www.aclpp.org
CA Dept of Health Services CLPPP	www.dhs.ca.gov/ps/deodc/childlead/index.htm
CA State Board of Equalization	www.boe.ca.gov/
Chicago Department of Public Health	www.ci.chi.il.us/Health/Lead.html
City of Philadelphia Law Department	www.phila.gov/law
Cleveland Department of Public Health	www.clevelandhealth.org/
CT Department of Social Services	www.dss.state.cs.us
Greensboro Engineering and Inspections Dept.	www.ci.greenboro.nc.us/eng.insp/default.htm
IA Department of Public Health BLPP	www.idph.state.ia.us/eh/lead_poisoning_prevention.asp
IN Dept. of Environmental Management	www.in.gov/idem
IN Family and Social Services Administration	www.in.gov/fssa/families/housing/index.html
Indianapolis Office of the Mayor	www.indygov.org/eGov/Mayor/home.htm
Kankakee (IL) Community Development Agency	www.ci.kankakee.il.us/cda.html
Los Angeles Housing Dept., Code Enforcement Bureau	www.ci.la.ca.us/LAHD
MA Dept. of Public Health CLPPP	www.mass.gov/dph/clppp/clppp.htm
MA Dept. of Revenue	www.massdor.com
MA Div. of Banks	www.mass.gov/dob
MA Div. of Insurance	www.mass.gov/doi
MA Div. of Professional Liscensure	www.mass.gov/dpl
Mahoning County Lead Hazard Control Program	www.mahoning-health.org
Manchester (CT) Health Dept.	http://humanservices.ci.manchester.ct.us/health
Marion County (IN) Health Dept. CLPPP	www.mchd.com/newlead.htm
MassHousing	www.masshousing.com/portal/server.pt
ME CLPPP	www.state.me.us/dhs/bohdcfh/led/index2.htm
ME Dept. of Health and Human Services	www.state.me.us/dhs
Milwaukee Health Dept. CLPPP	www.milwaukee.gov/display/router.asp?docid=2921

Milwaukee Health Dept. CLPPP	www.milwaukee.gov/display/router.asp?docid=2921
Montgomery County Community Development Office--Lead Hazard Control Program	www.co.montgomery.oh.us/Departments/com&econ/lead.html
National City Building and Safety Dept.	www.ci.national-city.ca.us/departments/building/Building1.htm
New Orleans Dept of Safety and Permits	www.cityofno.com/portal.aspx?portal=37
New Orleans Health Dept.	www.cityofno.com/portal.aspx?portal=48
NH Dept. of Health and Human Services CLPPP	www.dhhs.state.nh.us/DHHS/CLPPP/default.htm
NJ Dept. of Community Affairs	www.state.nj.us/dca/codes/bhi/index.shtml
NY State Energy Research and Development Authority	www.nyserda.org
Philadelphia Dept. of Health CLPPP	www.phila.gov/health/units/lead/index.html
Ramsey County (MN) Dept. of Public Health	www.co.ramsey.mn.us/PH/
RI Dept. of Health CLPPP	www.health.state.ri.us/lead/home.htm
RI Housing Resources Commission	www.hrc.ri.gov
Rocky Mount (NC) Planning and Development Dept.	www.ci.rocky-mount.nc.us/planning/main.html
St. Louis Affordable Housing Commission	http://stlouis.missouri.org/affordablehousingcommission/
San Francisco Dept. of Building Inspection	www.sfgov.org/site/dbi_index.asp
San Francisco Dept. of Health	www.dph.sf.ca.us/cehp/default.htm
VT Dept. of Health	www.healthyvermonters.info/
VT Housing and Conservation Board	www.vhcb.org/
WI Dept. of Health and Family Services CLPPP	http://dhfs.wisconsin.gov/lead/
Federal Government Agencies and Programs	
CDC--Childhood Lead Poisoning Prevention Program	www.cdc.gov/nceh/lead/lead.htm
EPA--Lead in Paint, Dust, and Soil	www.epa.gov/lead/
Head Start	www2.acf.dhhs.gov/programs/hsb/
HHS Children and Family Services	www.hhhs.gov/children/index.shtml
HUD--Office of Healthy Homes and Lead Hazard Control	www.hud.gov/offices/lead/
Medicaid	www.cms.hhs.gov/medicaid/mover.asp
Women, Infants, and Children	www.fns.usda.gov/wic/

State Nonprofits and Community-Based Organizations	
American Lung Association of Washington	www.alaw.org/
Baltimore Community Hist. and Archit. Preservation	www.ci.balitmore.md.us/government/historic/
Coalition to End Childhood Lead Poisoning	www.leadsafe.org
Connecticut Citizens Research Group	www.ccag.net/EnvHealth/HealthyHomes.htm
Environmental Health Coalition	www.environmentalhealth.org
Greater Minneapolis Day Care Association	www.gmdca.org/
Greensboro (NC) Housing Coalition	www.greensborohousingcoalition.com/Default
Improving Kids' Environment	www.ikecoalition.org
Lead Safe Pittsburg Coalition	www.leadsafepittsburgh.com/
Loyola University of Chicago School of Law ChildLaw Policy Institute	www.luc.edu/law/academics/special/center/child/special_progr-ams.shtml#childlawpolicy
Neighborhood Knowledge Los Angeles	http://nkla.sppsr.ucla.edu/index.cfm
New Jersey Citizen Action	www.njcitizenaction.org
New York City Coalition to End Lead Poisoning	www.nmic.org/nyccelkp.htm
NYPIRG	www.nypirg.org
Philadelphia Citizens for Children and Youth	www.pccy.org
Pratt Area Community Council	www.prattarea.org
Project 504 (MN)	www.project504.org
RI Childhood Lead Action Project	www.leadsafekids.org/programs.html
National Nonprofit Organizations	
Alliance for Healthy Homes	www.afhh.org
CEHRC	www.cehrc.org
National Center for Healthy Housing	www.centerforhealthyhousing.org
Media	
Detroit *Free Press*	www.freep.com/
Providence Journal	www.projo.com

APPENDIX C
LOCATIONS OF ILLUSTRATIONS

Location	Primary Actor	Building Block
California	California State Board of Equalization; California State Department of Health Services/California Childhood Lead Poisoning Prevention Branch	Impose Taxes or Fees on Polluters
California (Alameda County)	Alameda County Lead Poisoning Prevention Program	Hold Regular Lead-Safe Work Practices Trainings
California (Alameda County)	Alameda County Service Area, Joint Powers Authority, and Alameda County Lead Poisoning Prevention Program	Create a Special Real Estate Funding Mechanism
California (Alameda and Fresno counties)	CLPP Branch of CA Dept. of Health Services	Expand Lead Safety Education to Expectant and New Parents
California (Los Angeles)	Department of Housing	Secure Dedicated Funding for Code Enforcement
California (Los Angeles)	Los Angeles Healthy Homes Collaborative	Organize "Toxic Tours" for Policy Makers
California (Los Angeles)	Los Angeles Housing Department, Code Enforcement Bureau	Conduct Periodic Housing Code Inspections
California (Los Angeles)	Neighborhood Knowledge Los Angeles	Utilize Early Warning Systems for Deteriorating Properties
California (National City)	Environmental Health Coalition (EHC) and the Building and Safety Department	Teach Code Inspectors about Lead Safety through Joint Visits
California (San Francisco)	San Francisco Department of Public Health, Children's Environmental Health Promotion Program	Notify All Residents in a Building Found to Contain Lead Hazards
California (San Francisco)	San Francisco Department of Public Health, Childhood Lead Prevention Program (CLPP)	Require Agencies to Disseminate Lead Poisoning Prevention Information
California (San Francisco)	San Francisco Dept. of Building Inspection	Make the Most of Fines and Penalties

Location	Primary Actor	Building Block
Connecticut	Connecticut Department of Social Services	Home Assessments and Early Interventions for Families Served by Medicaid
Connecticut (Hartford)	Connecticut Citizens Research Group	Inform Landlords of Federal Lead Hazard Disclosure Requirements
Connecticut (Manchester)	Department of Health, Lead Abatement Project; Code Enforcement Unit	Make Lead Hazards a Violation of the Housing or Health Code
Connecticut (Manchester)	Manchester Health Department	Free Loans of Lead Safety Equipment
Illinois (Chicago)	Chicago Department of Public Health	Report Problem Landlords to HUD and EPA for Disclosure Enforcement
Illinois (Chicago)	Childhood Lead Poisoning Prevention Program (CLPPP) at the Chicago Department of Public Health	Connect Medicaid Data and Statewide Surveillance Databases
Illinois (Chicago)	Loyola University of Chicago School of Law ChildLaw Policy Institute	Compile State and Local Laws to Expedite Lead Safety
Illinois (Kankakee)	Kankakee Community Development Agency, Lead Poisoning Prevention Program	Equip Code Officials to Identify Lead Hazards and Pursue Enforcement
Indiana	Division of Family and Children, Housing and Community Service in the Department of Family and Social Services Agency	Adding Lead Safety to Weatherization and Training Programs
Indiana	Improving Kids' Environment (IKE) and the Lead-Safe Indiana Task Force	Publicize Restrictions on Unsafe Remodeling and Renovation
Indiana	Indiana Department of Environmental Management	Share Risk Assessment and Lead Sampling Services
Indiana	Indiana Department of Environmental Management (IDEM) & Family and Social Service Administration (FSSA) - Child Care Health Section	Incentives for Lead Safety in Child-Care Facilities
Indiana (Indianapolis)	Office of the Mayor	Publicize Problem Property Owners
Indiana (Indianapolis/-Marion County)	Childhood Lead Poisoning Prevention Program, Housing Division, Marion County Health Department, Marion County Health and Hospital Corporation	Consolidate Childhood Lead Poisoning Prevention and Code Enforcement Activities
Iowa	Iowa Department of Public Health Bureau of Lead Poisoning Prevention	Broadcast Lead Safety Training Widely

Location	Primary Actor	Building Block
Iowa (Dubuque)	Housing and Community Department	Equip Code Officials to Identify Lead Hazards and Pursue Enforcement
Louisiana (New Orleans)	Health Department and Department of Safety and Permits	Require Safe Work Practices During Remodeling, Repair, and Painting
Maine	Maine Department of Human Services	Perform Building-Wide Hazard Assessments in Multi-Unit Buildings Following Identification of Lead Hazards in One Troubled Unit
Maryland	Coalition to End Childhood Lead Poisoning	Establish a Lead-Safe Housing Registry
Maryland (Baltimore)	Baltimore City Commission for Historical and Architectural Preservation	Provide Local Property Tax Credits
Massachusetts	CLPPP, Massachusetts Dept. of Public Health	Expand Lead Safety Education to Expectant and New Parents
Massachusetts	Department of Public Health, Childhood Lead Poisoning Prevention Program	Screening Homes During Code Inspection
Massachusetts	Dept. of Public Health, Childhood Lead Poisoning Prevention Program; Dept. of Labor and Industries; Div. of Professional Licensure; Div. of Banks; Div. of Insurance	Impose Fees on Real Estate Transactions and Related Professional Licenses
Massachusetts	MassHousing	Establish a Revolving Fund to Stretch Dollars
Massachusetts	Department of Revenue	Offer an Income Tax Credit for Abatement
Michigan (Detroit)	Detroit Free Press	Use Investigative Journalism to Reveal the Dimensions of the Problem and Policy Shortcomings
Minnesota (Minneapolis)	Project 504	Enable Tenants and Community-Based Organizations to Take Action to Address Substandard Housing Conditions

Location	Primary Actor	Building Block
Minnesota (Minneapolis)	Project 504	Inform Rental Property Owners of Federal Lead Hazard Disclosure Requirements
Minnesota (Minneapolis and Hennepin County)	Greater Minneapolis Day Care Association	Collaborate for Lead Safety in Child Care Homes
Minnesota (Ramsey County)	Ramsey County Department of Public Health	Create Incentives to Integrate Lead Safety into Housing Rehabilitation
Minnesota (Ramsey County)	Ramsey County Department of Public Health	Expand Weatherization and Rehab Programs to Address Lead Safety
Missouri (St. Louis)	St. Louis Affordable Housing Commission	Create a Housing Trust Fund
New Hampshire	New Hampshire Department of Health and Human Services, Office of Community and Public Health, Childhood Lead Poisoning Prevention Program	Attach Lead Hazard Reduction Order to Property Deed
New Hampshire (Manchester)	The Way Home/Healthy Homes Services	Train and Employ Low-Income Community Residents in Hazard Control
New Jersey	Bureau of Housing Inspection	Require Rental Property Registration/Licensing
New Jersey	Department of Community Affairs, Division of Codes and Standards, Bureau of Housing Inspection	Secure Dedicated Funding for Code Enforcement
New Jersey	New Jersey Bureau of Housing Inspection	Conduct Periodic Housing Code Inspections
New Jersey (Newark)	New Jersey Citizen Action	Equip Community-Based Organizations and Service Providers
New York	New York State Energy Research and Development Authority	Access Electric Utility Public Benefit Funds
New York (Brooklyn)	Pratt Area Community Council	Use Data from Community Home Hazard Investigations to Advocate for Policy Solutions

Location	Primary Actor	Building Block
New York (New York City)	New York Public Interest Research Group (NYPIRG) and the New York City Coalition to End Lead Poisoning (NYCCELP)	Analyze and Publicize Data to Facilitate Improved Policies
New York (Rochester)	Orchard Street Community Health Center's Get The Lead Out Project	Create a "Demonstration Home" to Education Policy Makers and the Public
North Carolina (Greensboro)	Greensboro Housing Coalition	Engage Rental Property Owners on Lead Safety, Disclosure, and Other Responsibilities
North Carolina (Greensboro)	Greensboro Housing Coalition	Inform Rental Property Owners of Federal Lead Hazard Disclosure Requirements
North Carolina (Greensboro)	Greensboro Engineering & Inspections Department	Preclude Owners from Renting Units that have been Cited for Hazards
North Carolina (Rocky Mount)	Rocky Mount Planning and Development Department	Ensure that Do-It-Yourself Rehabbers are Trained
Ohio (Cleveland)	Cleveland Department of Public Health	Inform Rental Property Owners of Federal Lead Hazard Disclosure Requirements
Ohio (Cleveland)	Cleveland Childhood Lead Poisoning Prevention Program (CLPPP)	Adopt State and Local Lead Hazard Disclosure Laws
Ohio (Mahoning County)	Mahoning County Lead Hazard Control Program	Leverage Community Reinvestment Act for Lead Safety and Healthy Homes
Ohio (Montgomery County)	Montgomery County Community Development Office	Establish a Lead-Safe Housing Registry
Pennsylvania (Philadelphia)	City of Philadelphia Law Department; Court of Common Pleas; Department of Health's Inspections and Enforcement Division, Childhood Lead Poisoning Prevention Program	Create a Special Lead Court
Pennsylvania (Philadelphia)	Philadelphia Citizens for Children and Youth, Philadelphia Dept. of Health's Childhood Lead Poisoning Prevention Program	Analyze and Publicize Data to Facilitate Improved Policies

Location	Primary Actor	Building Block
Pennsylvania (Philadelphia)	City of Philadelphia Law Department, Health and Adult Services Unit	Abate Lead Hazards and Recover Costs When Owners Fail to Act
Pennsylvania (Pittsburgh/Allegheny County)	Lead Safe Pittsburgh Coalition	Create and Use Multi-Stakeholder Assessments and Reports to Advocate for Prevention
Rhode Island	Childhood Lead Action Project	Report Problem Rental Property Owners to HUD and EPA for Disclosure Enforcement
Rhode Island	Housing Resources Commission	Provide Technical Assistance to Property Owners
Rhode Island	Rhode Island Department of Health	Train Painters, Remodelers, and Maintenance Staff in Lead-Safe Work Practices
Rhode Island	Rhode Island Department of Health Childhood Lead Poisoning Prevention Program	Capitalize on Home Nursing Visits to Target Prevention Services
Rhode Island	Providence Journal	Use Investigative Journalism to Reveal the Dimensions of the Problem and Policy Shortcomings
Vermont	Vermont Department of Health	Certify Lead Sampling Technicians
Vermont	Vermont Department of Health, Childhood Lead Poisoning Prevention Program (CLPPP) and Vermont Social and Rehabilitative Services, Child Care Services Division.	Ensure Lead Safety in Licensed Child Care Programs
Vermont	Vermont Department of Health	Require an Inspection for Lead-Based Paint Hazards at Tenant Turnover
Vermont	Vermont Housing and Conservation Board	Require Rental Property Owners to Inform Tenants How to Report Deteriorating Paint

Location	Primary Actor	Building Block
Washington (King County)	American Lung Association of Washington	Assess and Address Multiple Hazards Simultaneously
Wisconsin	WI Department of Health and Family Services, Childhood Lead Poisoning Prevention Program	Consolidate and Analyze Data to Highlight Lead Poisoning "Hot Spots"
Wisconsin	Wisconsin Department of Health and Family Services, Childhood Lead Poisoning Prevention Program	Capitalize on Home Nursing Visits to Target Prevention Services
Wisconsin	Wisconsin Department of Health and Family Services, Childhood Lead Poisoning Prevention Program	Establish a Lead-Safe Housing Registry
Wisconsin (Milwaukee)	Milwaukee Health Department	Deploy Enforcement Orders and Grant Incentives in Tandem

APPENDIX D
ACRONYM INDEX

CAP—Community Action Program or Agency

CBO—Community-based Organization

CDBG—Community Development Block Grant program

CDC—U.S. Centers for Disease Control and Prevention

CEHRC—Community Environmental Health Resource Center

CLPPP—Childhood Lead Poisoning Prevention Program

CME—Continuing Medical Education

DOJ—U.S. Department of Justice

EBL—Elevated blood lead level

EPA—U.S. Environmental Protection Agency

FOIA—Freedom of Information Act

FTE—Full-time equivalent

GIS—Geographic Information Systems

HIPAA—Health Insurance Portability and Accountability Act of 1996

HUD—U.S. Department of Housing and Urban Development

ICC—International Code Council

LIHEAP—Low-Income Heating Energy Assistance Program

LPPP—Lead Poisoning Prevention Program

LST—Lead sampling technician

LSWP—Lead-safe work practices

NCHH—National Center for Healthy Housing

NIEHS—National Institute for Environmental Health Sciences

OHHLHC—HUD's Office of Healthy Homes and Lead Hazard Control

APPENDIX E
GLOSSARY OF TERMS

Abatement—Any set of measures designed to permanently eliminate lead-based paint or lead-based paint hazards. Abatement includes: (1) The removal of lead-based paint and dust-lead hazards, the permanent enclosure or encapsulation of lead-based paint, the replacement of components or fixtures painted with lead-based paint, and the removal or permanent covering of soil-lead hazards; and (2) All preparation, cleanup, disposal, and post-abatement clearance testing activities associated with such measures.

Clearance examination—An activity conducted following lead-based paint hazard reduction activities to determine that the hazard reduction activities are complete and that no soil-lead hazards or settled dust-lead hazards exist in the dwelling unit or worksite. The clearance process includes a visual assessment and collection and analysis of environmental samples.

Containment—The physical measures taken to ensure that dust and debris created or released during lead-based paint hazard reduction are not spread, blown, or tracked from inside to outside of the worksite.

Deteriorated paint—Any interior or exterior paint or other coating that is peeling, chipping, chalking or cracking, or any paint or coating located on an interior or exterior surface or fixture that is otherwise damaged or separated from the surface to which it was applied.

Dry sanding—Sanding without moisture; includes both hand and machine sanding.

Elevated blood lead level—The Centers for Disease Control and Prevention has established 10 micrograms per deciliter (μg/dL) or greater of lead in whole blood as an elevated blood lead level for children under age six.

Encapsulation—The application of a covering or coating that acts as a barrier between lead-based paint and the environment and that relies for its durability on adhesion between the encapsulant and the painted surface, and on the integrity of the existing bonds between paint layers and between the paint and the surface to which it was applied.

Environmental Health Perspectives (EHP)—A journal of the National Institute of Environmental Health Sciences (NIEHS) that presents peer-reviewed articles focused on the impacts of the environment on human health and often includes articles on childhood lead poisoning. *EHP* is an open access journal online at http://ehp.niehs.nih.gov/.

Feasibility of implementation—This section of the Building Blocks template estimates the ease in which a particular building block can be implemented. This section uses a feasibility scale that runs from low to variable to moderate to high to very high.

Federal Lead Hazard Disclosure law—A federal statute, administered by HUD and EPA, that requires owners of pre-1978 housing to disclose lead hazards to prospective tenants or buyers.

Friction surface—An interior or exterior surface that is subject to abrasion or friction, including, but not limited to, certain window, floor, and stair surfaces.

Hazard reduction—Measures designed to reduce or eliminate human exposure to lead-based paint hazards through methods including interim controls, abatement, or a combination of the two.

HEPA vacuum—A vacuum cleaner with an included high efficiency particulate air (HEPA) filter through which contaminated air flows. A HEPA filter is one that captures at least 99.97 percent of airborne particles of at least 0.3 micrometers in diameter.

Housing Choice Voucher Program (Section 8)—A HUD-administered assistance program that helps low-income families secure housing they may otherwise be unable to afford.

Impact surface—An interior or exterior surface that is subject to damage by repeated sudden force, such as certain parts of doorframes.

Interim controls—A set of measures designed to temporarily reduce human exposure or likely exposure to lead-based paint hazards. Interim controls include, but are not limited to, repairs, painting, temporary containment, specialized cleaning, clearance, ongoing lead-based paint maintenance activities, and the establishment and operation of management and resident education programs.

Key Partners—Those agencies, organizations, and individuals who work with or should be included in a given building block strategy. They are not the main parties responsible for implementation of a given building block.

Lead-based paint—Paint or other surface coatings that contain lead equal to or in excess of 1.0 milligram per square centimeter or 0.5 percent by weight.

Lead-based paint hazard—Any condition that causes exposure to lead from lead-contaminated dust, lead-contaminated soil, or lead-contaminated paint that is deteriorated or present in accessible surfaces, friction surfaces, or impact surfaces that would result in adverse human health effects as established by the CDC or another appropriate federal agency.

Lead-based paint inspection—A surface-by-surface investigation to determine the presence of lead-based paint and the provision of a report explaining the results of the investigation.

Lead-free housing—Target housing that has been found to be free of paint or other surface coatings that contain lead-based paint.

Lead-safe work practices (LSWP)—A collection of "best practices" techniques, methods, and processes, which minimize the amount of dust and debris created during remodeling, renovation, rehabilitation, or repair of pre-1978 housing. Lead-safe work practices help prevent the creation or exacerbation of lead-based paint hazards.

Lead Hazard Control Grant program—A HUD-administered program that awards grants to cities and states to facilitate the control of lead hazards, mainly in targeted low-income housing.

Lead hazard evaluation—A risk assessment, a lead hazard screen, a lead-based paint inspection, paint testing, or a combination of these to determine the presence of lead-based paint hazards or lead-based paint in a residential building.

Lead inspector—An individual trained under a state- or EPA-approved course to conduct official lead inspections. A lead inspector can also conduct clearance tests after abatement and non-abatement work as well as other lead sampling, but a lead inspector *cannot* perform a risk assessment. A lead inspector must attend three days of training to be certified.

Lead sampling technician—An individual trained under an EPA-approved course to conduct clearance testing after non-abatement work and to conduct other dust wipe sampling. A lead sampling technician *cannot* conduct a lead inspection or a risk assessment. A lead sampling technician must attend five and a half hours of training to be certified.

Paint stabilization—Repairing any physical defect in the substrate of a painted surface that is causing paint deterioration, removing loose paint and other material from the surface to be treated, and applying a new protective coating or paint.

Paint testing—The process of determining, by a certified lead inspector or risk assessor, the presence or the absence of lead-based paint on deteriorated paint surfaces or painted surfaces to be disturbed or replaced.

Painted surface to be disturbed—A paint surface that is to be scraped, sanded, cut, penetrated, or otherwise affected by rehabilitation work in a manner that could potentially create a lead-based paint hazard by generating dust, fumes, or paint chips.

Potential for replication—This section of the Building Blocks Template describes the ease in which jurisdictions may be able to implement a specific strategy described in a building block illustration. Such potential for replication is estimated using a standardized scale. The scale runs from low to moderate to high to very high.

Primary Actors—The main parties responsible for implementation of a given building block strategy. These can include public health departments, housing agencies, code enforcement agencies, and community-based organizations, among others.

Public health department—A state, tribal, county or municipal public health department, or the Indian Health Service.

Rehabilitation—The improvement of an existing structure through alterations, incidental additions, or enhancements. Rehabilitation includes repairs necessary to correct the results of deferred maintenance, the replacement of principal fixtures and components, improvements to increase the efficient use of energy, and installation of security devices.

Risk assessment—An on-site investigation to determine and report the existence, nature, severity, and location of lead-based paint hazards in residential dwellings, including: (1) Information gathering regarding the age and history of the housing and occupancy by children under age 6; (2) visual inspection; (3) dust wipe sampling or other environmental sampling techniques; (4) other activity as may be appropriate; and (5) provision of a report explaining the results of the investigation.

Risk assessor—An individual trained under a state- or EPA-approved course to conduct risk assessments. A risk assessor may also conduct paint inspections, clearance testing after abatement and non-abatement work, and other lead sampling. A risk assessor must attend five days of training to be certified.

Target housing—Any housing constructed prior to 1978, except housing for the elderly or persons with disabilities (unless any child who is less than 6 years of age resides or is expected to reside in such housing) or any 0-bedroom dwelling.

Visual assessment—Looking for, as applicable: (1) Deteriorated paint; (2) visible surface dust, debris, and residue as part of a risk assessment or clearance examination; or (3) the completion or failure of a hazard reduction measure.

Wet sanding or wet scraping—A process of removing loose paint in which the painted surface to be sanded or scraped is kept wet to minimize the dispersal of paint chips and airborne dust.

XRF device—A device that uses X-ray fluorescence technology to determine the lead content of paint. Official results from an XRF device can only be reported by a lead inspector or risk assessor.